ABC of
Pain

ABC series

An outstanding collection of resources – written by specialists for non-specialists

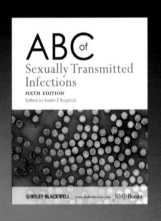

ABC of Sexually Transmitted Infections
SIXTH EDITION
Edited by Karen E Rogstad

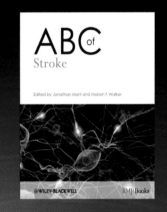

ABC of Stroke
Edited by Jonathan Mant and Marion F Walker

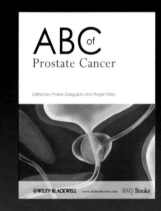

ABC of Prostate Cancer
Edited by Prokar Dasgupta and Roger Kirby

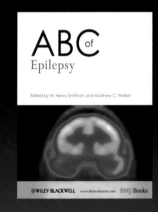

ABC of Epilepsy
Edited by W. Henry Smithson and Matthew C. Walker

The *ABC* series contains a wealth of indispensable resources for GPs, GP registrars, junior doctors, doctors in training and all those in primary care

▸ **Now fully revised and updated**

▸ **Highly illustrated, informative and a practical source of knowledge**

▸ **An easy-to-use resource, covering the symptoms, investigations, treatment and management of conditions presenting in day-to-day practice and patient support**

▸ **Full colour photographs and illustrations aid diagnosis and patient understanding of a condition**

For more information on all books in the *ABC* series, including links to further information, references and links to the latest official guidelines, please visit:

www.abcbookseries.com

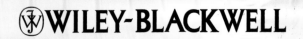

BMJ|Books

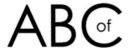

Pain

EDITED BY

Lesley A Colvin

Consultant Anaesthetist
Department of Anaesthesia, Critical Care & Pain Medicine
University of Edinburgh, Western General Hospital, Edinburgh, UK

Marie Fallon

St Columba's Hospice Chair of Palliative Medicine
Edinburgh Cancer Research Centre (CRUK)
University of Edinburgh, UK

WILEY-BLACKWELL
A John Wiley & Sons, Ltd., Publication

BMJ|Books

Library of Congress Cataloging-in-Publication Data
ABC of pain / edited by Lesley Colvin, Marie Fallon.
    p. ; cm. – (ABC series)
  Includes bibliographical references and index.
   ISBN 978-1-4051-7621-7 (pbk. : alk. paper)
   I. Colvin, Lesley, Dr. II. Fallon, Marie. III. Series: ABC series (Malden, Mass.)
   [DNLM: 1. Pain Management. WL 704]
   616′.0472 – dc23
                                              2011049095

Cover image: © iStockphoto.com/peepo
Cover design: Meaden Creative

A catalogue record for this book is available from the British Library.

Wiley also publishes its books in a variety of electronic formats. Some content that appears in print may not be available in electronic books.

Set in 9.25/12 Minion by Laserwords Private Limited, Chennai, India
Printed and bound in Malaysia by Vivar Printing Sdn Bhd

1   2012

Contents

Contributors

Jane C Ballantyne
Professor of Anesthesiology and Pain Medicine, UW Medicine Professor of Education and Research, Department of Anesthesiology and Pain Medicine, University of Washington, Seattle, WA, USA

James Campbell
Consultant in Orthopaedic Medicine, Department of Orthopaedics, Royal Infirmary of Edinburgh, Edinburgh, UK

Suzanne Carty
Consultant, Anaesthetic Department, Musgrove Park Hospital, Taunton, UK

Margaret Cullen
Consultant in Anaesthesia and Chronic Pain, Western General Hospital, Edinburgh, UK

Lesley A Colvin
Consultant/Senior Lecturer in Anaesthesia & Pain Medicine, Department of Anaesthesia, Critical Care & Pain Medicine, University of Edinburgh, Western General Hospital, Edinburgh, UK

Lesley Dickson
Clinical Nurse Specialist, Department of Anaesthetics, Critical Care and Pain Medicine, Western General Hospital, Edinburgh, UK

Paul Dieppe
Professor of Medical Education Research, Peninsula College of Medicine and Dentistry, Exeter, UK

Marie Fallon
St Columba's Hospice Chair of Palliative Medicine, Edinburgh Cancer Research Centre (CRUK), University of Edinburgh, UK

Susan Fleetwood-Walker
Chair of Sensory Neuroscience, Centre for Neuroscience Research, Veterinary Biomedical Sciences, Royal (Dick) School of Veterinary Studies, The University of Edinburgh, Edinburgh, UK

David Gillanders
Academic Director, Doctoral Programme in Clinical Psychology, University of Edinburgh, Edinburgh, UK

George R Harrison
Consultant in Pain Management and Anaesthesia, University Hospital Birmingham NHSFT and Honorary Senior Lecturer, Department of Pain Management, Queen Elizabeth Hospital Birmingham, Birmingham, UK

Dominic Hegarty
Consultant in Pain Management & Neuromodulation, Department of Anaesthesia and Pain Medicine, Cork University Hospital, Cork, Ireland

Mark I Johnson
Professor of Pain and Analgesia, Faculty of Health and Social Sciences, Leeds Metropolitan University and Leeds Pallium Research Group, Leeds, UK

Eija Kalso
Professor of Pain Medicine, University of Helsinki/Pain Clinic, Helsinki University Central Hospital, Helsinki, Finland

Anne MacGregor
Honorary Professor, Centre for Neuroscience & Trauma, Blizard Institute of Cell and Molecular Science, St Bartholomew's and the London School of Medicine and Dentistry, London, UK

Fiona MacPherson
Clinical Nurse Specialist Chronic Pain, Western General Hospital, Edinburgh, UK

James Maybin
Specialist Registrar, Anaesthesia, Glasgow Royal Infirmary, Glasgow, UK

Damien Murphy
Consultant in Anaesthesia and Pain Medicine, Department of Anaesthesia and Pain Medicine, Cork University Hospital, Cork, Ireland

Susan Nimmo
Consultant Anaesthetist, Department of Anaesthetics, Critical Care and Pain Medicine, Western General Hospital, Edinburgh, UK

Michael G Serpell
Consultant and Senior Lecturer, University Department of Anaesthesia, Glasgow University, Glasgow, UK

Blair H Smith
Professor of Population Science, Medical Research Institute, University of Dundee, Dundee, UK

Kimberley S Swanson
Department of Anesthesiology, University of Washington, Seattle, WA, USA

Nicola Torrance
Research Fellow, Medical Research Institute, University of Dundee, Dundee, UK

Carole Torsney
Caledonian Research Fellow, Centre for Neuroscience Research, Veterinary Biomedical Sciences, Royal (Dick) School of Veterinary Studies, The University of Edinburgh, Edinburgh, UK

Dennis C Turk
Department of Anesthesiology, University of Washington, Seattle, WA, USA

Suellen M Walker
Clinical Senior Lecturer in Paediatric Anaesthesia and Pain Medicine, University College London, Institute of Child Health and Great Ormond Street Hospital for Children, London, UK

Paul J Watson
Professor of Pain Management and Rehabilitation, University of Leicester, Leicester, UK

Debra K Weiner
Associate Professor of Medicine, Anesthesiology and Psychiatry, Geriatric Research, Education and Clinical Center, VA Pittsburgh Healthcare System and University of Pittsburgh School of Medicine, Pittsburgh, PA, USA

Joanna M Zakrzewska
Consultant in Oral Medicine, Oral Medicine, University College London Hospitals NHS Foundation Trust, London, UK

Preface

The aim of the wise is not to secure pleasure, but to avoid pain.

Aristotle

Regardless of the area of healthcare we work in, we will meet patients suffering from chronic pain. Pain can cause significant distress and suffering, with a major impact on patients' quality of life and on their families. Careful assessment and management of pain is an integral part of good clinical care, not something that should only be available through specialist teams. The field of pain management is expanding rapidly, with novel approaches to assessment techniques, improved understanding of the pathophysiology and developments in both pharmacological and non-pharmacological management strategies. While there are many excellent textbooks for specialists, there is however a need for a clear and concise evidence-based text, that provides an accessible introduction to this important area. This new title in the ABC series has gathered together a range of internationally recognised experts and practising clinicians to produce a book that we hope will prove of real practical value to primary care staff, trainee doctors, students and allied health professionals.

We have not set out to write a comprehensive text of all aspects of pain management but have attempted to include commonly seen chronic pain conditions, or in areas that may provide particular challenges. The first part of the book explores the epidemiology of pain, where it is clear just how common chronic pain is – something that has not been well-recognised until relatively recently. A clear outline of the basic science of pain mechanisms helps to provide a framework for understanding how chronic pain develops and how treatment may work. This section should also be helpful for students and junior doctors preparing for exams. As with any medical problem, a comprehensive but focused approach to pain assessment underpins any successful management plan, as outlined in the chapter from Prof Dennis Turk.

Subsequent chapters examine very common pain conditions, including musculoskeletal pain, neuropathic pain and also visceral pain, In these chapters we have suggested various approaches to assessment and management that we hope you will find useful. We then focus on pain in patient populations with particular needs, such as children, the elderly, those with drug dependency issues, cancer pain and also pain in pregnancy.

The final part of the book examines the wide range of therapies that can be used in the management of chronic pain. While this includes pharmacological management, including opioids, we have tried to consider the multidisciplinary strategies that are used successfully in the specialist setting and how these can be used in the non-specialist setting. Thus we have addressed psychological therapies, physiotherapy, and complementary therapies.

Each chapter has used illustrations and text boxes to highlight important points, aiding ease of reading and making it more accessible. For those interested in more details on a particular topic we have provided a further reading list, including useful web-based resources. Each chapter can be read in isolation, although you hope you will find the style persuades you to read chapters that might otherwise not appeal to you.

The specialist nature of complex pain management has been increasingly recognised over recent years, both by professional bodies such as the Royal College of Anaesthetists (London) with the establishment of a Faculty of Pain Medicine in April 2007, and also by politicians. The fact remains however, that the vast majority of pain problems are dealt with by non-specialists: it is essential that all healthcare professionals have the basic training and education required to enable them to confidently address pain problems and thus reduce suffering in our patients. We would like to thank all our contributors for their expert chapters and also their patience, as this book has taken some considerable time to reach fruition. Despite this, we hope that the end result is enjoyed by our readership, and that their patients reap the benefits of this.

Lesley A Colvin
Marie T Fallon

CHAPTER 1

Epidemiology of Chronic Pain

Blair H Smith and Nicola Torrance

Medical Research Institute, University of Dundee, Dundee, UK

OVERVIEW

- Chronic pain persists beyond normal wound healing, with around one in four adults suffering from chronic pain
- The majority of patients with chronic pain will be managed in the primary care setting, but complex cases will require specialist input
- Chronic pain, especially neuropathic pain, has a major impact on all aspects of general health
- Factors predisposing to chronic pain include those not amenable to intervention, such as increasing age and female gender, and also those that can be targeted, such as deprivation, or poor acute pain control
- Early identification and management of chronic pain are essential in order to minimise long term suffering and disability

Introduction

Pain is an individual experience, whose subjective nature makes it difficult to define, describe or measure, yet which is common to all human beings. As description and measurement are nonetheless essential, so, therefore, is a definition that suits both patients and professionals. Pain is helpfully, therefore, defined by the International Association for the Study of Pain (IASP) as *'an unpleasant sensory and emotional experience associated with actual or potential tissue damage, or described by the patient in terms of such damage'*.

Chronic pain is defined by the IASP as *'pain that persists beyond normal tissue healing time'*. A range of factors may be involved, including physical and biological factors, and also behavioural and cognitive factors, and these may dominate the experience of chronic pain, which is ultimately primarily subjective (Box 1.1).

Box 1.1 Acute and chronic pain

Acute pain	$\rightarrow \rightarrow \rightarrow \rightarrow \rightarrow \rightarrow$	Chronic pain
Physiological		*Pathological*
Health preserving		*Maladaptive*
Warns of damage		*Dysfunctional healing*
Allows evasive action		*Abnormal response to injury*

ABC of Pain, First edition. Edited by Lesley A Colvin and Marie Fallon.
© 2012 Blackwell Publishing Ltd. Published 2012 by Blackwell Publishing Ltd.

What is chronic pain?

There are many similarities in the symptoms and impact of chronic pain between most individuals who experience chronic pain, irrespective of its cause. Consequently, there are also many similarities in approaches to preventing or managing chronic pain of different aetiological or diagnostic backgrounds. This has led some to propose the existence of a 'chronic pain syndrome', and certainly for many clinical and research purposes, there is considerable merit in regarding chronic pain as a single, global, clinical entity (while also paying suitable attention to individual, treatable causes of chronic pain).

Why is epidemiology important?

Epidemiology is 'the study of the distribution and determinants of health-related states or events in specified populations *and the application of this study to control health problems'*.
   (Last RJ. (2001) *A Dictionary of Epidemiology*, 4th edn. Oxford: International Epidemiological Association.)

It is the latter part of this definition that makes it such an important science in clinical medicine. The last twenty or so years have seen the publication of many good quality epidemiological studies of chronic pain that have enhanced our understanding of its causes, impact and approaches to management. Good epidemiological research on chronic pain can, and does, provide important information on its classification and prevalence and factors associated with its onset and persistence. This can inform the design and targeting of treatment and preventive strategies (Box 1.2).

Box 1.2 How does epidemiology help us with chronic pain?

1 Identifies factors associated with chronic pain and those which lead to or favour chronicity
2 Aids development of interventions to prevent chronicity or to minimise its impact
3 Improving understanding of associated factors in development will inform the clinical management of the condition, thereby possibly limiting severity and minimising disability

4 Understanding how chronic pain impacts on quality of life and what associated factors have greatest adverse effect (e.g. physical, psychological or social)

5 Understanding the distribution of chronic pain can help to target appropriate management strategies at the subgroups most likely to benefit, and individuals with less severe chronic pain might be identified with a view to prevention of exacerbation

6 Evaluation of treatment strategies: Until the distribution, determinants, impact and natural history of chronic pain are understood, it is impossible to evaluate properly any intervention aimed at improving chronic pain

7 Allocation of health service resources: Ideally this should be informed by robust epidemiological data. With a condition of the importance of chronic pain, it is crucial that research information is available for health service planning

8 Allocation of educational resources: As with financial and clinical resources, appropriate education of professionals and patients can be greatly assisted by epidemiological study

Source: Adapted from Smith, BH, Smith, WC & Chambers, WA. (1996) Chronic pain – time for epidemiology. *Journal of the Royal Society of Medicine*, **89**, 181–183.

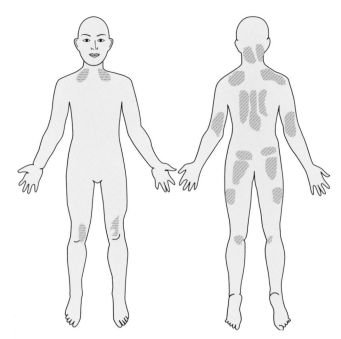

Figure 1.1 Pain diagram from patient with Chronic Widespread Pain.

How common is chronic pain?

The prevalence of chronic pain depends on exactly where, when and how it is measured. There is no universally agreed cut-off point between acute and chronic pain, but in the absence of other information, three months is often taken as the point beyond which 'normal tissue healing' should have taken place, and when pain therefore becomes chronic. Around one in four or five adults is currently experiencing chronic pain. A comprehensive literature review found a weighted mean prevalence of chronic pain of 25.9%. This is broadly similar to a large European study of over 46 000 people using a 6-month cut-off point (19.0%), and other systematic reviews.

Some studies have examined more severe, perhaps more clinically relevant, chronic pain. For example, 'chronic widespread pain' (bilateral pain above and below the waist, including the axial skeleton) has consistently been found to affect at least 5% of adults, and perhaps more than 11% (Figure 1.1).

A similar prevalence (5%) has been found for 'severe chronic pain' (intense, highly disabling, severely limiting pain). Pain with neuropathic features (which is often more severe and harder to treat than other pain) probably affects at least 6–8% of the population. These figures are similar to the prevalence rates of well-recognised conditions such as ischaemic heart disease and diabetes, for which health service resources are readily found. Chronic pain, however, generally attracts less attention and resource (perhaps because it is often regarded as a heterogeneous group of conditions, or as a symptom, rather than as a global entity requiring a global response) (Figure 1.2).

The commonest location of chronic pain is in the back, followed by the large joints (knee and hip). Other common causes of chronic

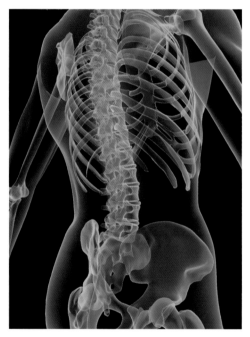

Figure 1.2 Chronic back pain is very common: around three out of four people will suffer from it at some point in their life. (Copyright © 2000, 2001, 2002 Free Software Foundation, Inc).

pain include headache, other joint pain, injury, and, importantly, neuropathic pain. The diagnosis of this is essential in order to initiate correct treatment (Chapter 6). In particular, persistent post-surgical pain (up to 30% of surgical patients experience pain beyond three months, and 5% experience severe chronic pain) may be under-recognised and, therefore, under treated. Additionally, most people (approximately 75%) with chronic pain report pain at more than one site, and 18% report it at five or more sites. Indeed, evidence suggests that it is the extent of chronic pain (i.e. the number of sites at which it occurs) that determines its impact (and therefore treatment required), rather than the specific cause or diagnosis. Furthermore, around 75% of people with chronic pain have had it for more than a year, and around half have had it for five years.

The impact of chronic pain

The duration and extent of chronic pain are relevant in considering its impact. There is a very strong association between the presence of chronic pain and poor general health, no matter how this is measured. Every dimension of health is worse in the presence of chronic pain, at a population level, compared with those who do not report chronic pain. There is a direct relationship between the severity of pain and poor health, with neuropathic pain being associated with the most adverse general health indicators. This includes physical, psychological and social aspects of health (Box 1.3). There is a strong link between chronic pain and depression, such that it frequently becomes impossible to separate the two: chronic pain without measurable depression is rare, and depression makes the presence of chronic pain much more likely. It is probable that there are common aetiological factors shared by chronic pain and depression.

Box 1.3 **Impact of chronic pain**

Chronic pain has an adverse impact on:

- Physical functioning
- General health
- Mental health
- Vitality
- Social functioning
- Emotional roles
- Mortality (further study needed)

Factors associated with chronic pain

While the prevalence of chronic pain tends to rise with age (at least to a certain age), some studies, however, report a lower prevalence in old and very old age groups. This phenomenon may be the result of a genuine reduction in prevalence (i.e. a protective effect of ageing), a survival effect or an artefact (i.e. older people not reporting chronic pain in surveys, thinking perhaps that is simply part of normal ageing); is the subject of current research. Cultural and geographical differences in the reported prevalence of chronic pain are also apparent, and have several potential and complex explanations (Box 1.4).

Box 1.4 **General factors associated with chronic pain**

- Female gender
- Increasing age
- Acute uncontrolled pain
- Deprivation
  - Household income
  - Level of education
  - Socio-demographic group

While we are unable reasonably to intervene on some biological and social risk factors for chronic pain identified by epidemiological research (age, sex, location and culture), other risk factors consistently reported are potentially amenable to intervention. Notable among these is the strong association between deprivation and the presence, extent and severity of chronic pain. This suggests that, whatever else is done to improve chronic pain, political support is required. The most imoprtant risk factor for chronic pain is *pain*, either acute pain, or chronic pain elsewhere in the body. This highlights the need for healthcare professionals to take all reports of pain seriously, addressing these to prevent future long-term ill health.

Early suggestions that the elimination of acute post-surgical pain minimises the risk of future chronic pain are encouraging, particularly if this can be extrapolated to other forms of acute pain. With other risk factors for chronic pain there is more variability but there are some that are potentially important for the design of interventions. Generally speaking, interventions based on these are at an early stage of design and evaluation, but the potential is there and the possible benefits great (Figure 1.3).

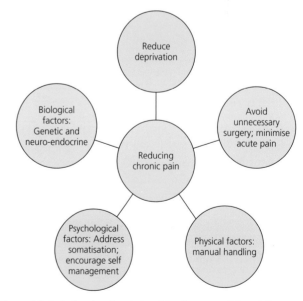

Figure 1.3 Reducing chronic pain by addressing some of the risk factors potentially amenable to intervention.

What is the cost of chronic pain?

The societal costs of chronic pain are difficult to gauge. One study of the economic burden of back pain in the United Kingdom estimated that it cost £10.7 billion, over than a decade ago. Some £1.6 billion of this was attributable to direct healthcare costs (the remainder being accounted for by lost productivity, benefits etc.; there is a demonstrable link between severity of chronic pain and the inability to remain or function in employment). It is estimated that around one in five consultations with a general practitioner (GP) is for a chronic pain-related reason, and that people with chronic pain consult their GP five times more frequently than those without.

Summary

In summary, therefore, chronic pain is a very common and important clinical condition, affecting individuals, the health services and society in diverse and adverse ways. The rest of this book explores some of the ways in which the problem can and must be addressed, and there is much good work currently underway to this effect in the clinical, educational and research arenas. This has been, and must continue to be, supported by epidemiological research, for 'one's knowledge of science begins when he can measure what he is speaking about and express it in numbers' (Lord Kelvin).

Further reading

Breivik, H, Collett, B, Ventafridda, V, Cohen, R & Gallacher, D (2006) Survey of chronic pain in Europe: Prevalence, impact on daily life, and treatment. *Eur J Pain*, **10**, 287–333.

Doth, AH, Hansson, PT, Jensen, MP & Taylor, RS (2010) The burden of neuropathic pain: a systematic review and meta-analysis of health utilities. *Pain*, **149** (2), 338–344.

Maniadiakis, N & Gray, A (2000) The economic burden of back pain in the UK. *Pain*, **84**, 95–103

McBeth J, Jones K. Epidemiology of chronic musculoskeletal pain. *Best Practice & Research in Clinical Rheumatology* **21**: 403–425, 2007.

Smith, BH & Torrance, N (2008) Epidemiology of Chronic Pain. In: McQuay, HJ, Kalso, E & Moore, RA (eds), *Systematic Reviews in Pain Research: Methodology Refined*. Seattle: IASP Press, pp. 247–273.

Smith, BH, Elliott, AM & Hannaford, PC (2004) Is chronic pain a distinct diagnosis on primary care? Evidence from the Royal College of General Practitioners Oral Contraception Study. *Family Practice*, **21**, 66–74.

Verhaak, PF, Kerssens, JJ, Dekker, J, Sorbi, MJ & Bensing, JM (1998) Prevalence of chronic benign pain disorder among adults: A review of the literature. *Pain*, **77**, 231–239.

CHAPTER 2

Pain Mechanisms

Carole Torsney and Susan Fleetwood-Walker

College of Medicine and Veterinary Medicine, The University of Edinburgh, Edinburgh, UK

OVERVIEW

- Chronic pain can occur following tissue injury or damage to the nervous system and, unlike acute pain, serves no useful function
- Injury modifies both peripheral and central components of the somatosensory nervous system, leading to misprocessing of sensory information and subsequent development of chronic pain syndromes
- Under normal conditions pain sensation is only evoked by painful stimuli; patients with chronic pain, however, may display pain sensation in the absence of sensory stimuli (*spontaneous pain*), exaggerated pain sensation to painful stimuli (*hyperalgesia*) and pain in response to touch (*allodynia*)
- Peripheral nervous system changes include heightened sensitivity of peripheral nerve terminals to sensory stimuli (*peripheral sensitisation*) and altered transmission of sensory signals to the spinal cord
- Central nervous system (spinal cord and brain) changes include distortion of spinal cord processing of sensory inputs, which increases spinal cord excitability and intensifies responses to sensory input (*central sensitisation*)
- These injury-induced changes are complex; they vary dependent on the type of injury, are influenced by factors such as genetic variability, and can also cause autonomic and affective changes

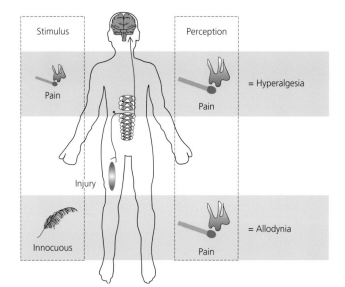

Figure 2.1 Chronic pain states arise following injury and are characterised by the symptoms of hyperalgesia (exaggerated pain), allodynia (touch-evoked pain) as well as continuing or spontaneous pain.

Introduction

Pain has its uses! It tells us to avoid situations that can cause serious damage to our bodies. That information is essential but when patients suffer from chronic, continuing pain it no longer serves any useful purpose and is an unpleasant and aversive experience.

Chronic pain states arise following tissue damage or injury to the peripheral and or central nervous system and are broadly termed 'inflammatory' or 'neuropathic', respectively. Both inflammatory and neuropathic pain states are characterised by spontaneous pain, hyperalgesia (exaggerated pain) and allodynia (touch evoked pain) (Figure 2.1). These symptoms may encourage behavioural adjustments that promote repair and recovery by limiting contact with,

for example, wounded tissue. However, if these symptoms persist beyond tissue healing, these chronic pain symptoms can be extremely debilitating and greatly reduce quality of life.

Chronic pain states transform dramatically the somatosensory nervous system, from one in which pain normally serves as a warning signal, promoting life and survival, to one in which pain is evoked by everyday activities and is counter-productive. In this chapter, those nervous system components that transduce and process sensory information are examined, how these components change or malfunction following injury is described and how these alterations are thought to produce chronic pain is explained.

Basic pain pathway

Sensory information is conveyed from the periphery to the central nervous system via primary sensory neurons. There are different types of sensory neurons (Table 2.1) but all have their cell bodies in the dorsal root ganglia (Figure 2.2).

ABC of Pain, First edition. Edited by Lesley A Colvin and Marie Fallon.
© 2012 Blackwell Publishing Ltd. Published 2012 by Blackwell Publishing Ltd.

Table 2.1 Some of the different types of peripheral nerve fibres.*

Fibre Type	Diameter (µm)	Conduction speed (ms⁻¹)	Function
Large myelinated			
Aα	12–20	70–120	Proprioception, motor
Aβ	5–12	30–70	Light touch, pressure
Small myelinated			
Aδ	2–5	12–30	Pain, cold, touch
B	<3	3–15	Preganglionic autonomic
Unmyelinated			
C	0.4–1.3	0.5–2	Pain, temperature, postganglionic sympathetics

*Adapted from Erlanger, J & Gasser, HS (1937) *Electrical signs of Nervous Activity*. Philadelphia, PA: University of Pennsylvania Press.

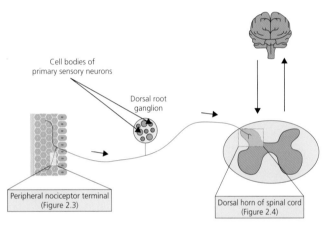

Figure 2.2 Basic somatosensory pathways. Sensory information is carried from the periphery to the spinal cord by primary sensory neurons, which have their cell bodies in dorsal root ganglia. Sensory information is then processed in the dorsal horn of the spinal cord before it is sent to the brain. There are also descending influences from the brain.

The pain-sensing primary sensory neurons, or 'nociceptors' have naked peripheral endings that terminate in the skin, mainly in the epidermal layer. These 'peripheral nociceptor terminals' possess an array of receptors or ion channels that transduce mechanical, thermal and chemical stimuli into neural signals (Figure 2.3a). Following sensory transduction, neural signals are then transmitted via primary sensory neurons to the dorsal horn of the spinal cord – the first stage of central processing of sensory input (Figure 2.4a).

The processing of sensory information within the dorsal horn is complex, involving local excitatory and inhibitory influences, as well as descending modulation from the brain. Importantly, this dorsal horn sensory processing determines which sensory signals are sent to higher centres to be perceived, where they may also influence emotional and autonomic function.

Chronic pain

Basic research focuses predominantly on animal models of pain states in the quest to comprehend the mechanisms underlying chronic pain. These include inflammatory, surgical nerve injury

and more sophisticated models in rodents that mimic pain conditions in the clinic (for example, demyelination, bone cancer, viral infection and arthritis). Analysis of these models reveals a multitude of changes, occurring within both peripheral and central sensory pathways, that are thought to underlie the misprocessing of sensory information leading to chronic pain. Chronic pain is essentially a pathological functioning of peripheral and central sensory pathways. It is recognised increasingly as a long term chronic condition in its own right, and might perhaps be considered as a chronic disease process.

Acute peripheral sensitisation

Inflammation or tissue injury releases a number of inflammatory mediators, for example prostaglandins, bradykinin, nerve growth factor, cytokines, adenosine triphosphate (ATP) and protons, from damaged tissue cells and inflammatory cells. Some directly activate nociceptors but many alter dramatically the sensitivity of nociceptors by activating intracellular signalling pathways, which can modulate transducer receptors locally and also ion channels in the sensory neurons that are crucial for the generation of neural signals (Figure 2.3b). This represents '*peripheral sensitisation*'. Local peripheral sensitisation mechanisms occur on a rapid timescale (a few minutes) allowing the somatosensory system to respond to tissue injury dynamically (Figure 2.5).

Chronic changes in peripheral sensitisation

Peripheral sensitisation also occurs over longer timescales by altering gene expression in nociceptors. Following sustained injury, the high levels of nociceptor activity and the binding of inflammatory mediators, such as NGF, to its receptor trigger signalling cascades that act to modify gene transcription in nociceptors. The resultant change in expression of transducer receptors and ion channels influences powerfully the flow of sensory information from the periphery to the spinal cord.

Peripheral sensitisation can trigger spontaneous pain

Chronic pain states are particularly difficult to treat when they involve damage to sensory nerves. The development of spontaneous or 'ectopic' activity in primary sensory neurons following peripheral nerve injury is thought to contribute importantly to neuropathic pain sensations such as spontaneous pain. Interestingly, ectopic activity is not limited to injured neurons but is observed in nearby intact sensory fibres, which also become hypersensitive. Ectopic activity is associated with altered expression and trafficking of ion channels, in particular sodium and potassium channels, that lead to an increased excitability of sensory neurons, such that neural activity can be generated spontaneously (Figure 2.6). There is much interest in sodium channel blocking agents as potential therapeutic agents, particularly for those subtypes ($Na_v1.8$ and 1.9) that are only expressed in the peripheral nervous system, for which agents should be devoid of central nervous system side effects.

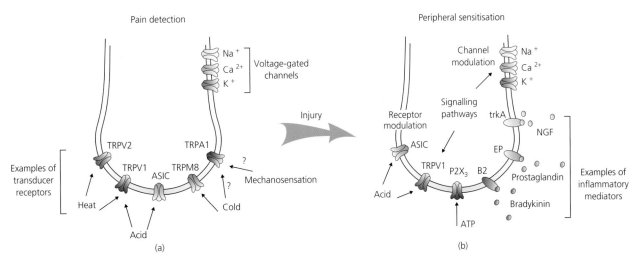

Figure 2.3 Pain detection by the peripheral nociceptor terminal and its amplification (peripheral sensitisation) in chronic pain states. (a) Noxious stimuli are transduced into electrical signals by specific receptors and ion channels. Our knowledge of pain detection has been transformed by the discovery of the TRP (Transient Receptor Potential) channels that are thermo- and chemo-sensitive. It is not fully understood which receptor or receptors are responsible for transducing mechanical pain. (b) Following injury, damaged tissue cells and inflammatory cells release inflammatory mediators. These activate intracellular signalling pathways that modify transducer receptor and ion channel function, which increases the sensitivity of the peripheral nociceptor terminal to sensory stimuli.

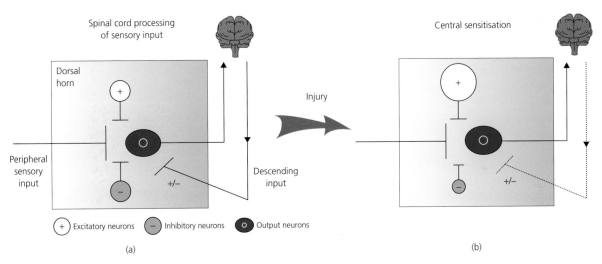

Figure 2.4 Representation of spinal cord processing of sensory input and its distortion (central sensitisation) in chronic pain states. (a) Incoming sensory information undergoes local and descending modulation in the spinal cord dorsal horn. (b) Dorsal horn sensory processing is distorted in chronic pain states. There is increased sensory input, increased local excitation, decreased local inhibition and altered descending control. Overall, this increases spinal cord excitability and amplifies responses to sensory input.

The resultant increased excitatory drive in peripheral sensory pathways evokes a complex array of changes within the central nervous system.

Central sensitisation

Central sensitisation was discovered in the early 1980s and was defined as an injury-induced increase in the excitability of the spinal cord that augments responses to sensory input. Subsequently, this activity-dependent plasticity has been shown to underpin inflammatory, neuropathic and other chronic pain states and is observed not only in the spinal cord, but also at higher levels (Figure 2.7).

Development of central sensitisation

Analogous to peripheral sensitisation, the early phase of central sensitisation, which is driven by sensitised and hyper-excitable peripheral pathways, involves activation of multiple receptors present on spinal cord neurons. These activate downstream signalling pathways that then phosphorylate ion channels and receptors and ultimately lead to an increase in spinal cord excitability. Later phases of central sensitisation (also like peripheral sensitisation) involve transcriptional changes and hundreds of genes undergo altered expression in the dorsal horn of the spinal cord following tissue or nerve injury. It is important to note that different types of injury generate distinct yet overlapping patterns of gene expression changes, suggesting that a similar wide ranging variety of therapeutics will be required for

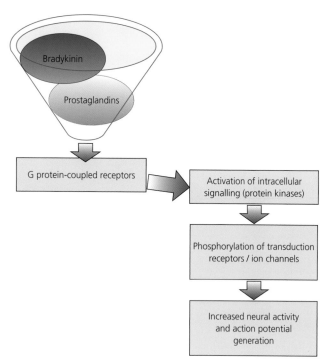

Figure 2.5 Example of factors leading to peripheral sensitisation.

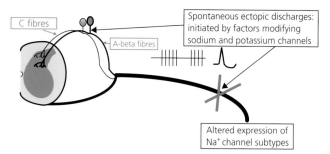

Figure 2.6 Peripheral factors leading to spontaneous pain after nerve injury.

effective treatment of chronic pain conditions. The central changes in chronic pain states combine to distort dramatically dorsal horn sensory processing (Figure 2.4b). Some of the key central changes are now outlined.

Increased excitability: changes in glutamate receptors

Spinal cord excitatory responsiveness is enhanced in chronic pain states. Both the excitatory α-amino-3-hydroxy-5-methyl-4-isoxazolepropionic acid (AMPA) and n-methyl-d-aspartate (NMDA) type glutamate receptors appear crucial to this process and show altered activity and expression patterns. The role of the NMDA receptor in chronic pain is well established, as early studies

showed that both the induction and maintenance of central sensitisation is NMDA receptor-dependent, highlighting the NMDA receptor as an obvious therapeutic target (Figure 2.8). However, because the NMDA receptor is widespread throughout the brain and spinal cord, NMDA receptor antagonists consequently may have a poor side effect profile as analgesics. Much effort is therefore being made to selectively target spinal NMDA receptors in chronic pain states. A subtype of AMPA receptor that is permeable to calcium has also been specifically implicated in chronic pain. Given the ubiquitous expression of both AMPA and NMDA type glutamate receptors, rather than directly blocking receptor activation another novel analgesic approach may be to target their adapter proteins, which are important for localisation and function of the receptors.

Decreased inhibitory activity

Spinal cord inhibitory control is also disrupted in chronic pain states. There are reduced levels of inhibitory neurotransmitters, such as glycine and gamma-aminobutyric acid (GABA), reduced inhibitory impact of their action on postsynaptic receptors and possibly even death of inhibitory spinal neurons. Interestingly, it has also been shown that inhibitory events can be converted into excitatory ones as a result of interactions between the immune system and central nervous system following nerve injury. Collectively these changes in inhibitory control will raise the net excitability in the spinal cord.

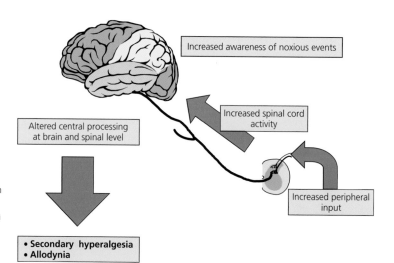

Figure 2.7 Features of central sensitisation. Whilst the phenomenon of peripheral sensitisation can explain heightened pain sensation at the site of injury (primary hyperalgesia), only central sensitisation can account for the spread of pain hypersensitivity outwith the site of injury (secondary hyperalgesia) and widespread touch-evoked pain (allodynia).

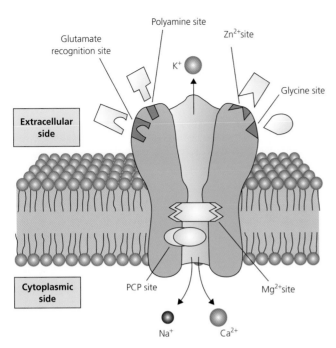

Figure 2.8 The NMDA receptor (reproduced with permission from Anaesthesia UK).

The immune system in central sensitisation

While it has long been established that immune cells are key players in peripheral sensitisation, the concept of central neuro-immune interactions is a relatively new and rapidly expanding area of research. Following injury, a subgroup of immune cells called microglia become activated in the spinal cord by agents released from primary sensory neurons that are damaged or dying. Microglia then release factors such as cytokines that regulate pain processing by modulating neuronal excitability. Given that these processes are only active in the injured state, this area looks promising in terms of potentially identifying novel analgesic targets, particularly since the immune system can be targeted, rather than the central nervous system. Other non-neuronal spinal cord cells that may play a role in some chronic pain states include astrocytes, with changes in astrocyte size and number in some chronic pain states (Figure 2.9).

Links between the spinal cord and the brain

Spinal cord neurons that send output signals to the brain have, not surprisingly, been shown to be required critically for chronic pain. Selective ablation of a specific group of spinal output neurons reduces significantly chronic pain symptoms in both inflammatory and neuropathic models. Interestingly, these output neurons are capable of retaining 'memory traces' of previous sensory input. These crucial output neurons target sites in the thalamus that project to the cortex and are also at the origin of a spinal cord–brain–spinal cord loop that is important for descending control of spinal cord excitability. These output neurons are thought to be important for chronic pain because they drive this loop, which controls spinal cord excitability and represents a key regulator of central sensitisation. In certain chronic pain states, regulation of spinal cord activity, via descending pathways from the brain, may switch from being

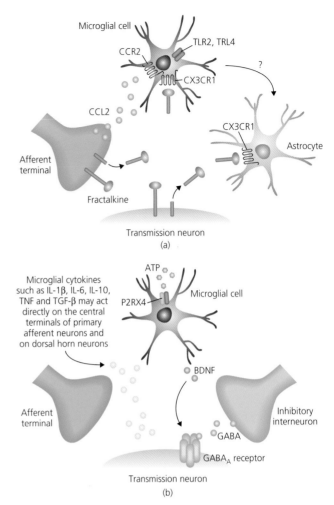

Figure 2.9 Role of spinal immune cells in pain processing. (a) Spinal microglial recruitment depends on signalling pathways involving Toll Like Receptor (TLR) 2 and TLR4, and on the chemokine CCL2 acting on CCR2. The neuronal protein fractalkine has a chemokine domain that can be cleaved from its membrane bound portion. Both bound and soluble fractalkine have chemokine function and may attract microglia as well as astrocytes by acting on CX3CR1. Because the microglial response to nerve injury precedes the proliferation of astrocytes, a direct path of communication may exist between these two glial cell types to coordinate their sequential temporal patterns of activation. (b) ATP binding to the purinergic receptor P2RX4 triggers microglial activation after nerve injury. Active microglia releases BDNF, which induces in a subpopulation of dorsal horn lamina I neurons an inversion of inhibitory GABAergic currents. In addition, microglial cytokines are likely to act directly on the central terminals of primary sensory afferents and on dorsal horn neurons.
(With permission, from Scholz, J & Woolf, CJ (2007) The neuropathic pain triad: neurons, immune cells and glia. *Nature Neuroscience*, **10**, 1361–1368).

predominantly inhibitory to excitatory, thus facilitating increased input from the spinal cord.

Summary

In conclusion, injury initiates a complex array of changes within both peripheral and central sensory pathways that manifest as chronic pain. Different types of injury produce very distinct, yet overlapping patterns of molecular and cellular changes and these are influenced further by gender, environmental, pyschosocial and genetic factors. This highlights the prevailing view that there will be no single analgesic that is perfect for all pain states. Ideally, treatment should be targeted at the underlying pathophysiological mechanisms and tailored to the individual to ensure successful management of these debilitating conditions.

Further reading

Devor, M (2006) Sodium channels and mechanisms of neuropathic pain. *J Pain*, **7**, S3–S12.

Garry, EM, Jones, E & Fleetwood-Walker, SM (2004) Nociception in vertebrates: key receptors participating in spinal mechanisms of chronic pain in animals. *Brain Res Brain Res Rev*, **46**, 216–224.

Mantyh, PW & Hunt, SP (2004) Setting the tone: superficial dorsal horn projection neurons regulate pain sensitivity. *Trends Neurosci*, **27**, 582–584.

Scholz, J & Woolf, CJ (2002) Can we conquer pain? *Nat Neurosci*, **5** (Suppl), 1062–1067.

Scholz, J & Woolf, CJ (2007) The neuropathic pain triad: neurons, immune cells and glia. *Nat Neurosci*, **10**, 1361–1368.

Woolf, CJ & Ma, Q (2007) Nociceptors-noxious stimulus detectors. *Neuron*, **55**, 353–364.

CHAPTER 3

Evaluation of the Patient in Pain

Dennis C Turk and Kimberly S Swanson

Department of Anesthesiology, University of Washington, Seattle, WA, USA

OVERVIEW

- Chronic pain is a complex problem with many interlinked facets that must be considered in an assessment
- The first essential step in managing chronic pain is a comprehensive assessment using a biopsychosocial perspective
- This process includes a comprehensive medical and physical assessment of the chronic pain patient
- The psychosocial assessment of the chronic pain patient is an important component of the overall assessment; while a detailed assessment may seem initially time consuming, it can be efficient in correctly directing therapy
- Self-report measures can be useful tools in the psychological assessment of a chronic pain patient

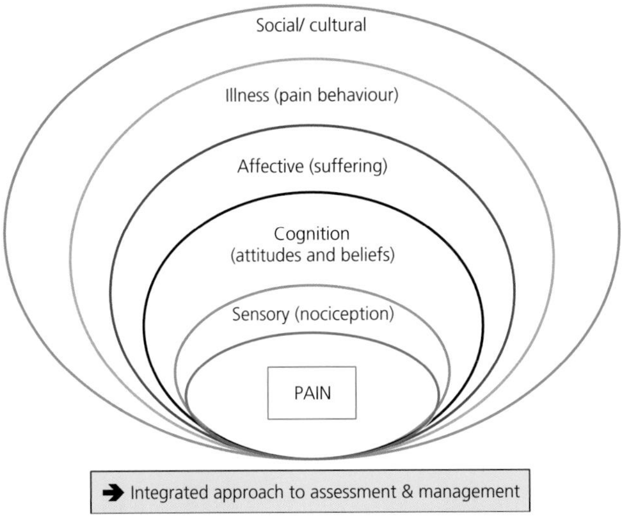

Figure 3.1 A biopsychosocial model of chronic pain. Many factors contribute to the pain experience and associated distress. These are closely inter-related: a dichotomous view of pain as being 'physical' or 'psychological' is not helpful.

The nature of chronic pain

The exact pathophysiology underlying many common pain problems (e.g. back pain, headache) is largely unknown. Conversely, 30% of *asymptomatic* individuals who reveal structural abnormalities on imaging studies suggestive of pain do not report pain. These observations suggest factors other than detectable physical pathology contribute to the report of pain. Thus, comprehensive assessment of the patient with chronic pain requires examination of psychosocial and behavioural factors as well as physical pathology (Figure 3.1).

The busy clinician may be concerned that a comprehensive assessment will require an excessive amount of time. There is no way around the problem. However, the assessment may be performed over several brief appointments and components involving patient completion of self-report questionnaires do not require clinician time beyond scoring and interpretation. The initial time for assessment may reduce the amount of time required throughout treatment.

Medical and physical evaluations

History and physical examination

Medical assessment of a patient with persistent pain begins with a current and past history and physical examination. In addition to

a general medical history, the healthcare provider should inquire in some detail about the pain (Figure 3.2). A physical examination should not only include a review of systems but also an assessment of physical functioning.

Laboratory testing and imaging procedures can rule out structural or biochemical abnormalities. However, physicians must not over-interpret either the presence or absence of objective findings unless they are consistent with the history and physical examination.

Psychological assessment

The healthcare provider should consider and evaluate the 'whole' patient, not just reported symptoms. Regardless of a documented organic cause for pain, the evaluation process can be helpful in identifying how biopsychosocial factors interact to influence the nature, severity, persistence of pain and disability, and response to treatment. This assessment is also helpful in treatment planning and anticipation of responses to treatment. General assessment considerations are illustrated in Box 3.1.

ABC of Pain, First edition. Edited by Lesley A Colvin and Marie Fallon.
© 2012 Blackwell Publishing Ltd. Published 2012 by Blackwell Publishing Ltd.

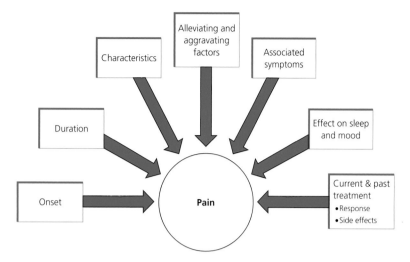

Figure 3.2 Important areas to cover when taking a pain history.

Box 3.1 **General assessment considerations**

Three central questions should guide assessment of people who report pain:

1 What is the extent of the patient's disease or injury (physical impairment)?
2 What is the magnitude of the illness? That is, to what extent is the patient suffering, disabled and unable to enjoy usual activities?
3 Does the individual's behaviour seem appropriate to the disease or injury or is there any evidence of amplification of symptoms for any of a variety of psychological or social reasons or purposes?

Interviews

Semi-structured interviews can be used to assess the myriad of psychosocial factors related to pain and disability. Not all patients require a detailed psychosocial evaluation. Outlined in Box 3.2 is a range of points that can be used as pre-screening questions with patients who report chronic pain and as a basis for determining whether a more thorough psychological evaluation is warranted.

Box 3.2 **Screening questions**

If there is a combination of more than six 'Yes' answers to the first 13 questions and 'No' to the last three questions, or if there are general concerns in any one area (e.g. substance abuse), a referral for a detailed psychological assessment should be considered.

1 Has the patient's pain persisted for three months or longer despite appropriate interventions and in the absence of progressive disease? [Yes]
2 Does the patient repeatedly and excessively use the healthcare system, persist in seeking invasive investigations or treatments after being informed these are inappropriate, or use opioid or sedative–hypnotic medications or alcohol in a pattern of concern to the patient's physician (e.g. escalating use)? [Yes]
3 Does the patient come in requesting specific opioid medication (e.g. dilaudid, oxycontin)? [Yes]

4 Does the patient have unrealistic expectations of the healthcare providers or the treatment offered (i.e. 'total elimination of pain and related symptoms')? [Yes]
5 Does the patient have a history of substance abuse or is he or she currently abusing mind altering substances? [Yes]
6 Does the patient display are large number of pain behaviours that appear exaggerated (e.g. grimacing, rigid or guarded posture)? [Yes]
7 Does the patient have litigation pending? [Yes]
8 Is the patient seeking or receiving disability compensation? [Yes]
9 Does the patient have any other family members who had or currently suffer from chronic pain conditions? [Yes]
10 Does the patient demonstrate excessive depression or anxiety? [Yes]. Straightforward questions such as, 'Have you been feeling down?' or 'What effect has your pain had on your mood?' can clarify whether this area is in need of more detailed evaluation.
11 Can the patient identify a significant or several stressful life events prior to symptom onset or exacerbation? [Yes]
12 If married or living with a partner, does the patient indicate a high degree of interpersonal conflict? [Yes]
13 Has the patient given up many activities (recreational, social, familial, in addition to occupational and work activities) due to pain? [Yes]
14 Does the patient have any plans for renewed or increased activities if pain is reduced? [No]
15 Was the patient employed prior to pain onset? [No] If yes, does he or she wish to return to that job or any job? [No]
16 Does the patient believe that he or she will ever be able to resume normal life and normal functioning? [No]

History of and current controlled- and illicit-substance use is important as some patients use opioid analgesics to manage their mood, and some have side effects that mimic the symptoms of depression (e.g. mood changes, altered sleep). Psychological dependence and aberrant behaviours related to prescribed pain-relieving medications and illicit drugs should be evaluated. A record of prescribed controlled substances and urine toxicology screening should be obtained and documented.

Referral for further evaluation may be indicated when the following are present:

- disability exceeding physical findings;
- disproportionate demands on the healthcare system;
- seeking medical tests and treatments when these are not indicated;
- significant emotional distress, addictive behaviours or continuing non-compliance with the treatment regimen.

A detailed outline of the areas addressed in a more extensive psychological interview for pain patients is contained in Box 3.3.

Box 3.3 **Areas addressed in psychological interviews**

Experience of pain and related symptom

- Location and description of pain (e.g. 'sharp', 'burning')
- Onset and progression
- Perception of cause (e.g. trauma, virus, stress)
- What has the patient been told about the symptoms and condition? Does the patient believe that this information is accurate?
- Exacerbating and relieving factors (e.g. exercise, relaxation, stress, massage)
- Pattern of symptoms (e.g. symptoms worse certain times of day or following activity or stress)
- Sleep habits (e.g. difficulty falling to sleep, maintaining sleep, or early morning wakening with inability to fall back asleep, and sleep hygiene)
- Thoughts, feelings, and behaviours that precede, accompany, and follow fluctuations in symptoms

Treatments received and currently receiving

- Medication (prescribed and over-the-counter). How helpful have these been?
- Pattern of medication use (as needed (PRN), time-contingent), changes in quantity or schedule
- Physical modalities (e.g. physical therapy). How helpful have these been?
- Exercise (e.g., Do they participate in a regular exercise routine? Is there evidence of deactivation and avoidance of activity due to fear of pain or exacerbation of injury?). Has the pattern changed (increased, decreased)?
- Complementary and alternative (e.g. chiropractic manipulation, relaxation training). How helpful have these been?
- Which treatments have they found the most helpful?
- Compliance/adherence with recommendations of healthcare providers
- Attitudes towards previous healthcare providers

Medical history

- What medical conditions does the patient currently have other than pain?
- What medical conditions has the patient had in past other than pain?

Compensation/Litigation

- Current disability status (e.g. receiving or seeking disability, amount, percentage of former job income, expected duration of support)
- Current or planned litigation

Responses by patient and significant others

- Typical daily routine
- Changes in activities and responsibilities (both positive and obligatory) due to symptoms
- Changes in significant other's activities and responsibilities due to patient's symptoms
- Patient's behaviour when pain increases or flares up
- Significant others' responses to behavioural expressions of pain
- What does the patient do when pain is not bothering him or her (uptime activities)?
- Significant other's response when patient is active
- Impact of symptoms on interpersonal, family, marital and sexual relations (e.g. changes in desire, frequency or enjoyment)
- Activities that patient avoids because of symptoms
- Activities continued despite symptoms. Pattern of activity and pacing of activity (can use activity diaries that ask patients to record their pattern of daily activities [time spent sitting, standing, walking and reclining] for several days or weeks)

Coping

- What does the patient do to cope with his or her symptoms?
- What role does the patient view himself or herself as having in symptom management?
- What are their current life stresses?
- What pleasant activities, if any, does the patient engage in?

Educational and vocational vistory

- What is the highest level of education completed, including any special training?
- What is the patient's work history, including military service?
- How long at most recent job?
- What were their thoughts and feelings about their most recent job and supervisor?
- What liked least and most about most recent job?
- Would the patient like to return to most recent job? If not, what type of work would the patient like?
- What is their current work status, including homemaking activities?
- What are their vocational and avocational plans?

Social history

- What is their current and past relationship with their family or origin?
- What is the history of pain or disability in family members?
- What is their marital history and current status?
- What is the quality of current marital and family relations?
- What is their current and history of friendships or social support outside family members?

Alcohol and substance use

- What is the current and history of alcohol use (quantity, frequency)?
- Has anyone ever expressed concerned about the patient's drug or alcohol use
- What is the history and current use of illicit psychoactive drugs?
- What is the history of substance abuse or prescription drug abuse in family members?
- History and current use of prescribed psychoactive medications

- What current and past prescription medications (i.e. opioids) are they taking and what are their patterns of use?

Psychological dysfunction

- Current psychological symptoms/diagnosis (depression including suicidal ideation, anxiety disorders, somatisation, post-traumatic stress disorder)
- Personal and/or family history of suicide attempts
- Is the patient currently receiving treatment for psychological symptoms? If yes, what treatments (e.g. psychotherapy or psychiatric medications). How helpful are the treatments?
- Personal and/or family history of psychiatric disorders and treatment including family counselling or hospitalisations for a psychiatric reason.
- History of or current, physical, emotional, and sexual abuse? If yes, was the abuse ever reported? What happened after the abuse was reported? Was the patient a witness to abuse of someone else?

Concerns and expectations

- Patient concerns/fears (e.g., Does the patient believe he/she has serious physical problems that have not been identified? Or that symptoms will become progressively worse and patient will become more disabled and more dependent? Does the patient worry that he or she will be told the symptoms are all psychological?)
- Explanatory models of pain held by the patient
- Expectations regarding the future and regarding treatment (will get better, worse, never change)
- Attitude toward rehabilitation versus 'cure'
- Treatment goal

Self-report assessment instruments

The most frequently used instruments for assessing pain are: the McGill Pain Questionnaire (MPQ), Beck Depression Inventory (BDI) and Multidimensional Pain Inventory (MPI). These instruments are not alternatives to interviews; rather, they may uncover or confirm issues to be addressed in more depth. Standardised instruments are easy to administer, require less time for the healthcare provider than extensive interviews, assess a wide range of behaviours, obtain information about behaviours that may not be reported or that are unobservable, can be analysed for reliability and validity, and may have control data available to compare responses from the patient to a larger population.

Pain intensity

Pain is inherently subjective, thus self-report provides the gold standard in assessments of pain and its characteristics. Several methods are used to evaluate current pain intensity – numerical scale (NRS) (Figure 3.3), verbal ratings scales (VRS), and visual analogue scales (VAS). Each of the methods appears reliable and valid. No one method is consistently superior in detecting improvements associated with pain treatment. However, there are important differences among these measures. Patients tend to prefer NRS and VRS measures over VAS measures. VAS measures demonstrate more missing data than do NRS measures. Other measures are available to assess

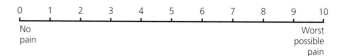

Figure 3.3 Rating scales can be useful, with good patient compliance with numerical rating scales (NRS). 0 = no pain; 1 – 3 = mild pain; 4 – 6 = moderate pain; 7 – 10 = severe pain.

pain in children and those who are unable to communicate verbally or to understand NRS, VRS, and VAS measures.

Pain quality

The efficacy of treatment varies potentially for different pain qualities (e.g. throbbing vs. electric-shock like). Thus, pain quality may identify treatments that are efficacious for certain types of pain but not for overall pain intensity. The Short-Form McGill Pain Questionnaire (SF-MPQ) assesses sensory and affective pain descriptors and its sensory and affective subscales have demonstrated responsiveness to treatment in a number of clinical trials.

Assessment of overt expressions of pain

In addition to self-reports of pain, behaviours (e.g. limping, moaning) are surrogates for pain. These behaviours are observable and indicate how patients communicate their pain and distress. Responses by significant others, including healthcare providers, to these overt expressions of pain influence the frequency with which these behaviours are elicited. Healthcare providers should also consider patients' healthcare use, statements by significant others and observational methods to quantify systematically various behavioural manifestations of pain and note the factors that increase or decrease them (e.g. attention, activity).

Assessment of emotional distress

Emotional distress is prevalent in people with chronic pain and an assessment challenge. Symptoms such as fatigue, appetite change, sleep disturbances, weight changes and decreased libido often associated with pain are also characteristic of depressive disorders. Therefore, improvements or deterioration in such symptoms can reflect changes in pain, emotional distress, or both. The BDI provides a well-accepted criterion of the level of psychological distress and responses to treatment. Anxiety is also commonly observed in patients with chronic pain. Healthcare providers should inquire about patients' fears, worries and emotional arousal. Standardised questionnaires are available to assess anxiety (e.g. the Pain Anxiety Symptom Questionnaire).

Assessment of function

Self-report measures have been developed to assess a range of functional activities. There are a number of well-established, generic disease-specific and pain-specific measures of functional status. Disease-specific measures are designed to evaluate the impact of a specific condition that may be more sensitive to the effects of treatment on function. However, generic measures provide information about physical functioning and treatment benefits that can be compared across different conditions. Self-report measures of physical functioning have been shown to be highly associated with actual physical functioning.

Secondary gain

Because the report of pain is often not accompanied by objective pathology, there is frequently an implicit assumption that pain in the absence of physical evidence is motivated by an attempt to receive some benefit, commonly referred to as secondary gain, such as monetary payment, avoidance of undesirable activity, or attention. Although secondary gain may be relevant, it is rarely the sole cause of symptoms. The absence of objective physical pathology and desire for disability compensation are not sufficient to assume that a patient is malingering. The healthcare provider should balance all of the factors obtained in the evaluation before assuming that reports of pain are exclusively the result of the desire to obtain some positive outcome.

Assessment of coping and psychosocial adaptation to pain

Historically, psychological measures designed to evaluate psychopathology (e.g. the Minnesota Multiphasic Personality Inventory, MMPI) have been used to identify individual differences associated with reports of pain, even though these measures were usually not developed for or standardised on samples of medical patients. Because disease status and medication can affect responses, patients' scores may be elevated; therefore, responses to these measures should be interpreted with caution. A number of measures have been developed for use specifically with pain patients (e.g. MPI, Brief Pain Inventory (BPI)).

Conclusions

Pain is a complex, idiosyncratic experience. Assessment and treatment of pain can be complicated by the web of influential factors that modulate the overall pain experience and report of pain and associated disability. Furthermore, traditional biomedical approaches with diagnostic tests are often inconclusive because structural damage and persistent pain complaints do not coincide. Pain research has shown repeatedly that pain is not just a physiological phenomenon, and that a range of 'person variables', such as psychosocial, environmental and behavioural factors, plays a significant role in determining the occurrence, severity and quality of pain. Adequate assessment requires a comprehensive overview of the pain experience and its impact on the patient. Medical and psychological assessments may include a range of self-report inventories that can be used in conjunction with interviews and medical examinations. An adequate pain assessment means the evaluation of the entire person with chronic pain, including their prior medical and psychosocial history, and within their social context rather than just focusing on pathology or the primary complaint. Such an understanding of the person and not just the patient is necessary in order to develop and execute a successful treatment plan.

Acknowledgement

Preparation of this manuscript was supported in part by grants from the National Institute of Arthritis and Musculoskeletal and Skin Diseases (AR47298) awarded to the first author.

Further reading

Battie, MC & May, L (2001) Physical and occupational therapy assessment approaches. In: Turk, DC & Melzack, R (Eds) *Handbook of pain assessment*, 2nd edn, pp. 204–224. New York: Guilford Press.

Beck, AT, Steer, RA, Ball, R & Ranieri, WF (1996) Comparison of Beck Depression Inventories -IA and -II in Psychiatric Outpatients. *Journal of Personality;* **67**, 588–597.

Cleeland, CS & Ryan, KM (1994) Pain assessment: global use of the Brief Pain Inventory. *Annals of Academic Medicine*, **23**, 129–138.

Hadjistavropoulos, T, von Baeyer, C & Craig, KD (2001) Pain assessment in persons with limited ability to communicate. In: Turk, DC & Melzack, R (Eds) *Handbook of pain assessment*, 2nd edn, pp. 134–152. New York: Guilford Press.

Keefe, FJ, Williams, DA & Smith, SJ (2001) Assessment of pain behaviors. In: Turk, DC & Melzack, R (Eds) *Handbook of pain assessment*, 2nd edn, pp. 170–190. New York: Guilford Press.

Kerns, RD, Turk, DC & Rudy, TE (1985) The West Haven-Yale Multidimensional Pain Inventory (WHYMPI). *Pain*, **23**, 345–356.

McCracken, LM, Zayfert, C & Gross, RT (1992) The Pain Anxiety Symptoms Scale: development and validation of a scale to measure fear of pain. *Pain*, **50**, 67–73.

Melzack, R (1975) The McGill Pain Questionnaire: major properties and scoring methods. *Pain*, **1**, 277–299.

Melzack, R (1987). The short-form McGill Pain Questionnaire. *Pain*, **30**, 191–197.

Turk, DC & Melzack, R (Eds.) (1992/2001) *Handbook of pain assessment*, 1st/2nd edns. New York, Guilford.

CHAPTER 4

Chronic Musculoskeletal Pain

Paul Dieppe

Peninsula College of Medicine and Dentistry, Exeter, UK

OVERVIEW

- The majority of chronic pain experienced by older adults is musculoskeletal in origin
- The symptom experience and impact of this pain varies greatly
- Chronic musculoskeletal pain is often associated with reduced activity, sleep disturbance, fatigue and mood alterations, and can result in severe disability
- Regional pain in a single joint area is very common. It may be referred from above, or be due to periarticular lesions, as well as arthritis. A good history and careful examination should result in an accurate diagnosis
- There are two main forms of arthritis: osteoarthritis (OA) and inflammatory arthritis. Pain in OA does not correlate well with pathology, is largely 'mechanical' in nature, and is difficult to treat. The pain of inflammatory arthritis is associated with severe joint stiffness and responds well to anti-inflammatory therapy
- Generalised musculoskeletal pain in the absence of peripheral pathology ('fibromyalgia') is also common. There is evidence that this condition is due to pain sensitisation and loss of the normal inhibitory mechanisms that help reduce pain

---

Introduction

Musculoskeletal pain is ubiquitous – everyone gets it. There are three main causes:

1. everyday activities that put unusual or repetitive strains on the system;
2. acute traumatic events;
3. musculoskeletal diseases.

Everyone is familiar with the aches and pains that generally follow unaccustomed activity and most of us will have had at least one episode of acute post-traumatic pain affecting our muscles, bones or joints. These problems are generally short lasting and not very bothersome. However, huge numbers of us, particularly older adults, also experience chronic, intrusive musculoskeletal pain. Recent surveys suggest that 30–50% of older adults suffer chronic

pain, most of which comes from the musculoskeletal system. The spine is the commonest site involved (Back pain is dealt with in Chapter 5) followed by the knees, shoulders and feet. A disease is not always apparent, but of the chronic musculoskeletal disorders that cause chronic pain osteoarthritis is by far the most common.

Although some diseases, such as gout, are renowned for the severe acute, self-limiting pain that they can cause, this chapter only covers chronic musculoskeletal pain and disease.

The anatomy and physiology of musculoskeletal pain

Figure 4.1 shows a diagrammatic representation of a synovial joint and its surrounding structures. The articular cartilage is aneural, but the other structures are all richly innervated, with particularly dense sensory innervation seen at the insertions of tendons or ligaments into bone (the entheses), the subchondral bone and the periosteal covering of bones. Nociceptive systems seen in these structures include the A-delta fibres responsible for acute sharp pain, and the C fibres responsible for chronic dull, throbbing pains (Chapter 2). Sensory input from these structures is an essential part of our function – as we stand or walk the entheses are 'sensing' the strain arising from the different muscles and joints, and through spinal pathways adjusting muscle tone accordingly, without our being aware of anything. Normally, these everyday activities, including more strenuous things such as running, do not excite the pain systems, but it now appears that in joint disease, particularly if inflammation is present, the system can become sensitised such

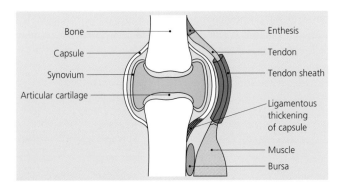

Figure 4.1 Cross-section of a synovial joint and surrounding tissues marking the most richly innervated structures.

ABC of Pain, First edition. Edited by Lesley A Colvin and Marie Fallon.
© 2012 Blackwell Publishing Ltd. Published 2012 by Blackwell Publishing Ltd.

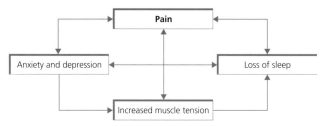

Figure 4.2 People with chronic pain often get into a 'viscious circle' of problems. The pain leads to anxiety and depression, which can make the pain worse, as well as affecting sleep. Lack of sleep also increases pain. Muscle tension is increased by pain, and can also lead to more pain as well as contributing to further loss of sleep, anxiety and depression.

that normal everyday activities become painful. In addition, pain sensitisation can occur at the spinal level, and cortical activity can lead to disinhibition of musculoskeletal pain.

The experience of musculoskeletal pain

Healthcare professionals and academics carrying out research on musculoskeletal pain have focused their attention almost entirely on the *severity* of musculoskeletal pain, with some additional emphasis on whether it occurs at night or not. So, the 'patient' is asked how bad the pain is and whether it wakes them at night or not, and management strategies are suggested accordingly. However, it is clear that those with chronic musculoskeletal pain can experience a rich and varied set of symptoms not adequately described by enquiries about pain severity. It is now known, for example, that people with osteoarthritis usually experience two quite different sorts of pain – their 'usual' activity-related dull ache, and unpredictable attacks of severe, short lasting, more bothersome pain; and people with inflammatory rheumatic diseases experience severe morning stiffness in joints, which may be their overriding symptom.

Nearly everyone with chronic musculoskeletal pain, be it back pain, fibromyalgia or due to osteoarthritis or rheumatoid arthritis, also experiences four other associated problems:

1 activities limitations due to pain (with associated lack of participation in life);
2 sleep disturbance;
3 fatigue;
4 mood disturbance.

The interactions between sleep problems, fatigue, anxiety/depression and pain are complex and not fully understood. The interactions can work in both directions (pain causing depression and depression increasing pain for example), and it is clear that some people can get into a 'viscious circle' in which loss of sleep, fatigue and anxiety or depression increase the amount of pain experienced, with the pain also causing sleep and mood problems (Figure 4.2).

A classification of musculoskeletal disease and pain

The WHO classification of musculoskeletal disorders breaks them into five groups, which, in rough order of frequency in the population, are shown in Figure 4.3.

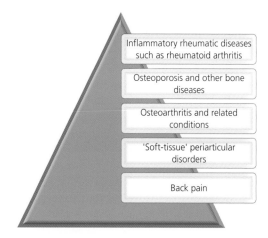

Figure 4.3 WHO classification of musculoskeletal disorders.

A recent 'paradigm shift' in the approach to musculoskeletal (and other) diseases has been the recognition that pain should be thought of as a separate issue – the 'fifth vital sign in medicine' and a disease in its own right. In that context the tendency is to classify chronic musculoskeletal pain according to its site(s) of origin – it may be localised to a single joint (such as a shoulder or knee), to a region or limb (the back or the legs for example) or it may be generalised pain (often considered synonymous with fibromyalgia).

Some aspects of regional conditions, arthritis, and fibromyalgia are discussed briefly here.

Regional pain and the 'soft-tissue' periarticular disorders

If someone presents with chronic pain at a single joint site there are three possible causes:

1 The pain is referred from a more proximal site in the body. The classic musculoskeletal example of this is hip disease presenting with knee pain (Figure 4.4). Other examples include spinal problems being referred to the arm or leg, and, of course, cardiac problems being referred to the arm. It is essential to examine the structures 'above' the affected joint as well as the painful area itself when trying to make a diagnosis of the cause of regional musculoskeletal pain. An additional point to note is that localised tenderness can be referred from above, rather than indicating that the local tissue under the examiners' fingers is diseased.

2 The pain comes from the periarticular 'soft tissues' surrounding the joint There are several structures around the joint which can cause pain. The entheses, referred to above are a common cause, small tears in the structures giving rise to inflammation and pain associated with point tenderness at the anatomical site and pain reproduced by putting strain on the affected ligament or tendon. Common examples are lateral or medial epicondylitis at the elbow (tennis or golfer's elbow, respectively), achilles tendonitis, and 'policeman's heel' (plantar fasciitis). Problems in the body of the ligament or tendon can also occur, as in some forms of achilles tendonitis, and most commonly at the shoulder, where

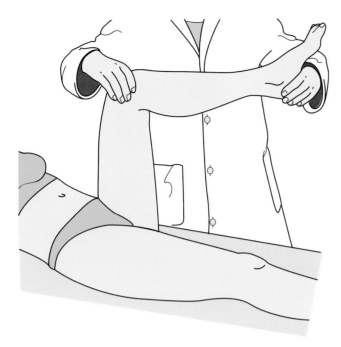

Figure 4.4 Examining the hip to make sure that the subject's knee pain does not come from the hip.

the tendons of the rotator cuff are often damaged. Problems can also occur with bursae surrounding joints (subacromial bursitis at the shoulder or trochanteric bursitis at the hip for example), in which case there is swelling of the bursa (which may be visible if superficial, as in olecranon bursitis of the elbow – 'boozer's elbow', but may only be detectable with imaging techniques such as ultrasound) (Figure 4.5). Other causes of periarticular problems include inflammation of tendon sheaths (as in 'trigger finger' for example), muscle injuries or localised nerve compression (as in carpal tunnel syndrome).

3 The pain is caused by intra-articular problems – arthritis There are two main sorts of intra-articular disorder – mechanical and

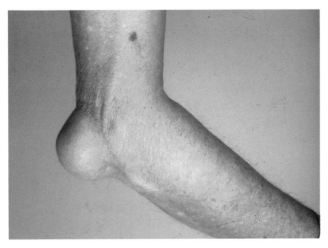

Figure 4.5 Olecranon bursitis. Note the huge fluid-filled swelling over the olecranon process of the elbow. Pain can arise from pressure in the bursa caused by the build up of fluid from the inflamed synovial lining of the bursa.

inflammatory. Mechanical problems may be due to traumatic damage to an intra-articular structure, such as a knee meniscus, or to osteoarthritis. Unsurprisingly mechanical joint problems are characterised by mechanical symptoms and signs – such as 'locking' of a joint or crepitus on examination, while the inflammatory disorders are characterised by warmth and swelling of the affected joints. There are a large number of inflammatory conditions of joints, as mentioned in the next section.

In general, a careful examination can reveal the cause of regional 'joint' pain, and many of the disorders mentioned above are referred to as 'easily curable rheumatism', as they can be alleviated by simple, logical approaches, such as taking the stress off an affected enthesis, or injecting local steroid to get rid of focal inflammation in a bursa.

Arthritis

A detailed description of the many different types of arthritis and their characteristics is obviously beyond the scope of this chapter.

Osteoarthritis (OA) is a very common condition of older adults; it is characterised by focal areas of loss of articular cartilage associated with subchondral bone change in synovial joints. It affects hands, knees and hips most often (as well as the spine), and may be accompanied by local soft-tissue periarticular problems or by fibromyalgia, making the pain problem difficult to sort out and treat. Radiographs are used to diagnose the disease (Figure 4.6) but are of little value in management and should not be used routinely. OA pain is largely use-related and often described as a deep 'ache', sometimes interrupted by spasms of a more severe and different form of pain. Pain often disturbs sleep. Short-lasting stiffness of joints after inactivity is usually reported as well. Pain management in OA is difficult, but is well summarised in a recent National Institute for Health and Clinical Excellence (NICE) report that stresses the need for an holistic approach, with prominent use of

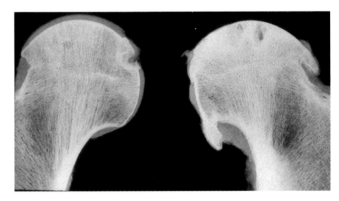

Figure 4.6 Osteoarthritis of the hip. These slab radiographs are of the femoral head from a normal hip (left) and from a hip with severe osteoarthritis (right). The normal hip has a smooth, rounded shape to the femoral head, and the bone is covered with a thin layer of articular cartilage. The osteoarthritic femoral head has lost most of the cartilage, the bone has become flattened and misshapen, and there are large bony outgrowths at the margins of the joint (osteophytes). Note the changes in the bone below the damaged cartilage – these include areas of thickening of the bone (sclerosis) and cysts. Much of the pain in osteoarthritis may be generated in the abnormal, active subchondral bone.

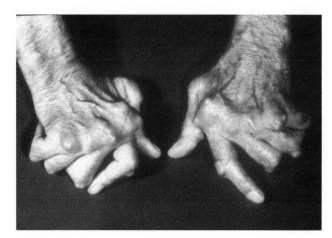

Figure 4.7 Rheumatoid arthritis. The hands of a patient with advanced rheumatoid arthritis. Note the muscle wasting associated with disuse of the joints, the joint deformity caused by joint destruction and the rheumatoid nodules in the subcutaneous tissue over the joints. Paradoxically, hands at this stage of the disease may cause much less pain than in the earlier, more inflammatory phase of the condition.

non-pharmacological therapy; there is no effective treatment for the OA disease process other than joint replacement.

Inflammatory arthritis can be caused by several different diseases, most of which are most common in young adults. They include rheumatoid arthritis (RA), the sero-negative spondarthritides (such as ankylosing spondylitis or psoriatic arthritis), crystal-related arthritis, infections of joints and connective tissue diseases. Most of these diseases are characterised by unrelenting inflammation of the synovial lining of joints, bursae and tendon sheaths. RA is the commonest condition and it has a fairly strong female bias; it usually presents with pain, and swelling of the small joints of the hands and feet; this moves to more proximal joints with time and over a period of many years the inflammation may become less intense, but joint damage, due to erosion of cartilage and bone, can become severe (Figure 4.7). Prominent features of the pain of RA include severe stiffness in the mornings (it may take someone several hours to get washed and dressed in the morning) and fatigue. The pain itself is usually described as fairly constant and severe, and although it has some relationship to use of the joints, this is not generally as strong a feature as it is in people with OA. The pain of RA responds better to anti-inflammatory therapy than it does to analgesics. The management of RA has improved hugely over the last two decades and if early antirheumatic therapy, with agents such as methotrexate or anti-TNF therapies, is used the condition can usually be well controlled.

Fibromyalgia

Fibromyalgia is a common condition of middle-aged adults (more common in women than men), characterised by widespread musculoskeletal pain, devastating fatigue and sleep and mood disturbances. It has overlaps with chronic fatigue syndrome, irritable bowel syndrome and migraine, and features of these conditions may accompany the dominant musculoskeletal pain and fatigue. Tender spots are commonly present in a number of well defined sites (Figure 4.8).

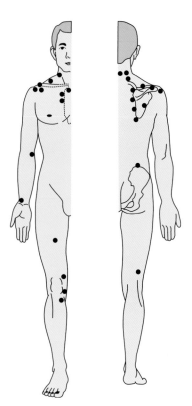

Figure 4.8 Sites of tenderness in fibromyalgia.

There is no peripheral pathology apparent in the muscles, joints or periarticular tissues to explain fibromyalgia. There are, however, a number of risk factors and associated phenomena that suggest that is likely to be due to central sensitisation or disinhibition of pain pathways. The risk factors include genetic and family influences, other psychosocial factors and environmental triggers including stress and infections. The associations include other painful conditions (including headache, which is very common) and disturbances of pain thresholds (with abnormal sensitisation and allodynia both being common), autonomic nervous system activity and neuroendocrine function. Fibromyalgia is a difficult condition to manage. Pharmacological approaches include the use of centrally acting agents including antidepressants and pregabalin; non-pharmacological approaches include exercise-based interventions and cognitive behavioural therapy.

Further reading

Graven-Nielsen, T & Arendt-Nielson, L (2010) Assessment of mechanisms in localized and widespread musculoskeletal pain. *Nat Rev Rheumatol*, **6**, 599–606.

Graven-Nielsen, T, Arendt-Nielson, L & Mense, S (Eds) (2008) *Fundamentals of Musculoskeletal Pain*. Seattle, WA: International Association for the Study of Pain.

Kidd, BL (1999) What are the mechanisms of regional musculoskeletal pain? *Ballieres Best Pract Res Clin Rheumatol*, **13**, 217–230.

Linton, S (Ed.) (2002) *New Avenues for the Prevention of Chronic Musculoskeletal Pain*. Elsevier.

MacKichan, F, Wylde, V & Dieppe, P (2008) The assessment of musculoskeletal pain in the clinical setting. *Rheum Dis Clin North Am*, **34**, 311–330.

CHAPTER 5

Management of Low Back Pain

James Campbell[1] and Lesley A Colvin[2]

[1]Department of Orthopaedics, Royal Infirmary of Edinburgh, Edinburgh, UK
[2]Department of Anaesthesia, Critical Care & Pain Medicine, Western General Hospital, University of Edinburgh, Edinburgh, UK

OVERVIEW

- Low back pain is extremely common and infrequently has serious underlying pathology
- A small, but significant, percentage of people affected by back pain develop a chronic problem with associated disability
- Appropriate early diagnosis and management reduces disability
- The evidence for effectiveness of injection therapies is limited, but selected patients may benefit from appropriate interventions
- Although total resolution of pain is often not possible, a key aim of management is to avoid chronicity and encourage effective self management

---

Introduction

While the majority of adults will have suffered from back pain at some point in their life, it is usually a minor self-limiting condition. Pain in the lower back is extremely common: around 60% of the adult population can expect to have a back problem at some time in their life. Although most back pain is generally benign a significant percentage of the population will develop chronic pain and disability (Box 5.1). The vast majority of adults with low back pain are labelled as having 'mechanical low back pain', which implies that there is a problem with the mechanism of the back for which a generic treatment package is probably appropriate in the first instance.

Box 5.1 **Low back pain and disability**

- 3–4% of young adults (below are 45) are chronically disabled by low back pain
- 5–7% of older adults (45+ years) are chronically disabled by low back pain

---

The mechanical problem may be structural (e.g. disc pathology, facet joint arthropathy), but frequently is a 'mechanical

dysfunction', where the normal mechanism is disturbed. Recognising this possibility (dysfunction vs. pathology) is central to managing patients and their expectations. With some persistent chronic pain states the recognition that the functional disturbance is central may require a further shift in our treatment paradigm.

Mechanical dysfunction

The most important first step in management of a patient with back pain is to rule out serious pathology without unnecessary investigations (Figure 5.1). Low back pain is a symptom not a disease. The main thrust of medical education is to recognise pathology, so when we are presented with a symptom (low back pain) that has a low probability of having a pathological basis we may struggle to deal with our uncertainty and possibly patient demands for scans (Table 5.1).

Start by considering the 'red flags' – pointers to possible pathology that may indicate the need for investigation (Box 5.2).

Box 5.2 **Red flags**

- Age <20 or onset >55 years
- Trauma
- Constant, progressive, non-mechanical pain
- Previous history of carcinoma, systemic steroids, drug abuse, HIV
- Systemically unwell/weight loss
- Persisting severe restriction of lumbar flexion
- Widespread neurology
- Structural deformity
- Cauda equine syndrome
- Inflammatory pain – night pain, morning stiffness

Guidelines

Many back pain guidelines have been published in several countries. Generally, the content of these guidelines is similar. The Cochrane Back Group has reviewed the published evidence for many aspects of back pain. In general, there is a paucity of high

---

ABC of Pain, First edition. Edited by Lesley A Colvin and Marie Fallon.
© 2012 Blackwell Publishing Ltd. Published 2012 by Blackwell Publishing Ltd.

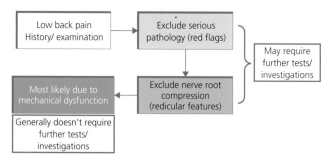

Figure 5.1 Initial approach to managing low back pain.

Table 5.1 Common features associated with mechanical low back pain compared to nerve root pain.

Mechanical back pain	Nerve root pain
• Presentation usually aged 20–55 • Pain in lumbosacral region, buttocks and thighs • Pain mechanical in type – varying with activity and time • Patient otherwise well	• Unilateral leg pain worse than back pain • Pain usually radiates to foot • Numbness and paraesthesia • Nerve irritation signs • Motor, sensory or reflex change

Table 5.2 Suggestions for diagnosis and treatment of low back pain.

Summary of recommendations for diagnosis of low back pain	Summary of recommendations for treatment of low back pain
• Diagnostic triage (non-specific LBP, radicular syndrome, specific pathologic change) • History taking and physical examination to exclude red flags • Physical examination for neurologic screening (including straight leg raising test) • Consider psychosocial factors if there is no improvement • Radiographs not useful for non-specific LBP.	• Reassure patients (favorable prognosis) • Advise to stay active • Prescribe medication if necessary (preferably time contingent): paracetamol, non-steroidal anti-inflammatory agents, consider muscle relaxants or opioids • Discourage bed rest • Consider spinal manipulation for pain relief • Do not advise back-specific exercises **Chronic pain** • Refer for exercise therapy

quality, well designed trials, often making it difficult to evaluate truly the effectiveness of various therapies. Several guidelines focus on acute low back pain (up to an arbitrary 12 weeks). In the United Kingdom further guidelines were published by The National Institute for Health and Clinical Excellence (NICE) in 2009 specifically for the patient group with persistent back pain from 6 weeks to 12 months (http://www.nice.org.uk/CG88). For example, surgical intervention for appropriately selected patients suffering from lumbar disc prolapse with radicular features does reduce the acute attack more quickly than conservative management, but may have a limited effect on the long-term natural disease history (Table 5.2).

Investigations – how valuable is Magnetic Resonance Imaging (MRI)?

Plain radiographs of the lumbar spine have a limited role (unless there is a 'red flag' indication), and all published guidelines recognise this. However, there may be an expectation from patients that an MRI scan is necessary to assess their problem and there may be some pressure to refer for this. Unless there is nerve root pain an MRI scan is unlikely to be helpful. The high rate of abnormal findings in both discs and joints in the normal population makes the interpretation of any positive results problematic (Figure 5.2). It is essential to consider the clinical presentation alongside any MRI findings.

Facet joint degeneration is also common in the general population. In a cadaveric study (and hence no knowledge of subject symptoms) facet joint changes were almost universally found. Twin studies suggest that physical loading specific to occupation and sport has a minor role in disc degeneration, and that genetic factors explain 75% of the variance.

Accordingly the relationship between anatomical changes and symptoms of low back pain remains controversial.

Acute, chronic and recurrent pain

Not only is low back pain a vague symptom with multiple possible causes, but also patient characteristics change according to the duration and past history of their symptoms. Management of acute back pain is essentially different from that of chronic back pain. Keefe has suggested a number of potential key features in the development of chronic back pain (Figure 5.3).

Treatment options

All possible treatments can be considered under the four headings of (i) pharmacological, (ii) psychological, (iii) surgical and (iv) physical. It is logical that a mechanical disturbance might benefit from a mechanical (physical) treatment, and because physiotherapy has been part of the National Health Service for historical reasons

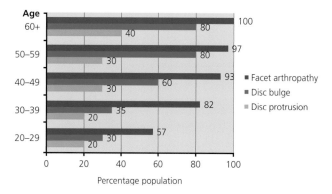

Figure 5.2 A range of 'positive' findings on MRI scan may be found in the normal adult population. (Adapted from: Jensen, MC, Brant-Zawadzki, MN & Obuchowski, N (1994) Magnetic resonance imaging of the lumbar spine in people without back pain. *N Eng J Med*, **331** (2), 69–73).

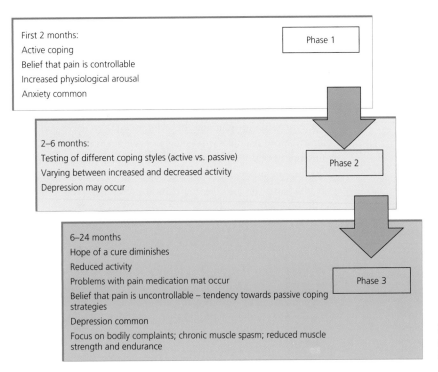

First 2 months:
Active coping
Belief that pain is controllable
Increased physiological arousal
Anxiety common

Phase 1

2–6 months:
Testing of different coping styles (active vs. passive)
Varying between increased and decreased activity
Depression may occur

Phase 2

6–24 months
Hope of a cure diminishes
Reduced activity
Problems with pain medication mat occur
Belief that pain is uncontrollable – tendency towards passive coping strategies
Depression common
Focus on bodily complaints; chronic muscle spasm; reduced muscle strength and endurance

Phase 3

Figure 5.3 Potential features seen in development of chronic low back pain. (Adapted from Keefe and Blumenthal, 1982).

in the United Kingdom, back pain has traditionally been managed by 'referral to physiotherapy'. However, physiotherapy is a profession that encompasses a range of treatments and it is also one of three physical therapy professions, along with osteopathy and chiropractic.

Manipulation

Consideration of manual therapy is included in many of the guidelines for acute pain, and in the NICE guidelines for lower back pain from 6 weeks to 12 months, it is recommended offering manual therapy for up to 9 sessions over 12 weeks. Not all physiotherapists offer manual therapy but both osteopathy and chiropractice are professions regulated by statutory bodies that can be accessed by patients (Chapter 17.)

Acupuncture

The NICE guidelines also suggest offering up to 10 sessions of acupuncture needling over a 12-week period. Although the evidence base may be questioned, it is extremely safe and relatively cheap, and is a useful treatment modality for pain relief (Chapter 19, Figure 19.1).

Injections

Various interventional pain procedures have been used to help back pain. They are used generally for chronic pain when non-invasive strategies have been ineffective. Although the NICE guidelines advise specifically against injections, this view has been challenged. A recent Cochrane review concluded that, while good quality trials are lacking, there is likely to be a selected subgroup of patients, with subacute and chronic back pain, which will benefit from injection therapy (Chapter 16).

Psychology

The biopsychosocial model of pain (Figure 5.4) reflects the potential role of non-physical factors that may contribute to chronic pain, including back pain. Some of these factors can be addressed using psychological techniques (Chapter 15).

Some of the risk factors that may predispose to developing chronic pain syndromes are seen in chronic back pain (Table 5.3), and may require expert psychological intervention to enable the patient to progress with effective self management.

The development of chronicity certainly adds to the complexity of the problem (Box 5.3), the following management principles being suggested (adapted from Sharpe and Wessley (1997) Non-specific ill

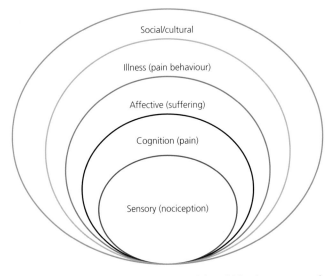

Social/cultural

Illness (pain behaviour)

Affective (suffering)

Cognition (pain)

Sensory (nociception)

Figure 5.4 The Biopsychosocial Model: a useful model for the treatment of chronic back pain.

Table 5.3 Risk factors predisposing to chronic back pain and long-term disability.

- Pain duration >2 years + multiple surgical interventions
- A past history of:
  - prolonged recovery from similar or other types of pain
  - physical, emotional or sexual abuse
- Job dissatisfaction
- Low levels of activity, excessive pain behaviours, and solicitous or exceptionally punitive family members' responses to such behaviours
- Fear-avoidance with negative fear-based beliefs about pain and activity
- Pre-morbid anxiety, distress or depression
- Somatization

(Adapted from: Manek, NJ &MacGregor, AJ (2005) Epidemiology of back disorders: prevalence, risk factors and prognosis. *Curr Opin Rheumatol*, **17**(2), 134–140; and Eimer, BN& Freeman, A (1998)*Pain management psychotherapy – a practical guide*. New York: John Wiley & Sons, Inc.)

health: a mind-body approach to functional somatic symptoms. In: *Mind-Body Medicine, a clinician's guide to psychoneuroimmunology* (Ed. A Watkins). Edinburgh: Churchill Livingstone, 169–186).

1 make the patient feel understood;
2 establish a positive collaborative relationship;
3 correct misconceptions about disease and give a positive explanation of symptoms;
4 avoid unnecessary investigation and treatment;
5 negotiate a formulation and treatment plan with the patient.

Box 5.3 **The 'six dysfunctional Ds' of chronic pain syndromes (as described by Eimer and Freeman*) are as follows:**

1 emotional **d**istress (e.g. anxiety, conflict, anger, hostility, resentment, alienation)
2 behavioural and cognitive **d**eficits
3 varying degrees of **d**isability related to work
4 **d**epression
5 physical **d**e-conditioning
6 **d**isturbed sleep

*Eimer, BN& Freeman, A (1998) *Pain management psychotherapy – a practical guide*. New York: John Wiley & Sons, Inc.

Central Sensitivity Syndrome (CSS)

Chronic low back pain may be a manifestation of 'central pain' and lie on the spectrum of central sensitivity syndromes that includes fibromyalgia, irritable bowel syndrome, chronic fatigue and many others (Table 5.4). There is evidence from epidemiology, twin studies and functional imaging to suggest that chronic central pain is itself a disease that may manifest itself in different body areas but with similar underlying mechanisms.

Features of central hypersensitivity include:

- core symptoms: multifocal pain, fatigue, insomnia, psychological and cognitive or memory problems;
- the occurrence and the severity of these symptoms occur in a wide range of the population;

Table 5.4 Spectrum of chronic pain syndromes. Chronic low back pain may, in some circumstances, be a central pain syndrome.*

Peripheral (nociceptive)	Neuropathic	Central (non-nociceptive)
Primarily due to inflammation or mechanical damage in periphery	Damage or entrapment of peripheral nerves	Primarily due to a central disturbance in pain processing
NSAID & opioi dresponsive; may respond to procedures	Responds to both peripheral and central pharmacological therapy	Tricyclic anti depressants; neuroactive compounds most effective
Behavioural factors-minor	Behavioural factors - variable	Behavioural factors - more prominent
Examples: Osteoarthritis; rheumatoid arthritis; cancer pain	Examples: Post herpetic neuralgia; diabetic neuropathy; persistent post surgical pain	Examples: Fibromyalgia; irritable bowel syndrome; tension headache; Idiopathic low back pain

*(see Ablin, K&Clauw, DJ(2009) From Fibrositis to Functional Somatic Syndromes to a Bell-Shaped Curve of Pain and Sensory Sensitivity: Evolution of a Clinical Construct,*Rheum Dis Clin N Am*, **35**, 233–251.)

- current diagnostic labels are at some level arbitrary as there is no objective tissue pathology to confirm or discriminate the disease process;
- symptoms and syndromes occur approximately twice as commonly in women than men, and there is a strong familial predisposition;
- many different stress factors may trigger or exacerbate these symptoms and syndromes;
- similar types of therapies are efficacious for all of these conditions, including pharmacologic (e.g. tricyclic compounds such as amitriptyline) and non-pharmacologic treatments (e.g. exercise and cognitive behavioural therapy). Conversely, individuals with these conditions typically do not respond to therapies that are effective when pain is due to damage or inflammation of tissues (e.g. non-steroidal anti-inflammatory drugs, opioids, injections, surgical procedures).

Apart from tricyclics, serotonin-noradrenaline reuptake inhibitors (such as duloxetine and tramadol) and alpha-2-delta ligands (such as gabapentin and pregabalin) can be effective for central sensitivity. However, any one of these classes of drug will tend only to help around one third of patients.

Conclusion

Patients with the symptom of pain in the lumbar region present a considerable challenge in terms of both diagnosis and treatment. The largest diagnostic category, mechanical pain, is itself heterogeneous, comprising different dysfunctions and different pathologies that remain difficult to characterise with current investigations. It is the heterogenicity of subjects that tends to confound the clinical trials assessing current treatments. For example, there is no doubt some low back pain arises from the sacroiliac joint but the specificity and sensitivity of diagnostic tests, including CT arthography remains uncertain. There has been a successful movement away from the 'injury' model of back pain but the 'mechanical dysfunction' that can cause acute back pain and the 'central sensitivity syndrome' that can develop in the chronic situation are perhaps not yet fully embraced.

Further reading

Battie, MC, Videman, T & Parent, E (2004) Lumbar disc degeneration: Epidemiology and genetic influences. *Spine*, **29** (23), 2679–2690.

Clarke, A, Jones, A, O'Malley, M & Robert McLaren, R (Eds) (2009) *ABC of Spinal Disorders*. John Wiley & Sons Ltd. ISBN 978-1-4051-7069-7.

Cochrane Back Review Group; frequently updated review of the evidence for back pain management: http://www.cochrane.iwh.on.ca/. Recent relevant reviews include:Gibson, JNA & Waddell, G (2011) Surgical interventions for lumbar disc prolapse. Cochrane Database of Systematic Reviews. 2 (Art. No.: CD001350). DOI: 10.1002/14651858.CD001350.pub4. Staal, JB, de Bie, R, de Vet, HCW, Hildebrandt, J & Nelemans, P (2008) Injection therapy for subacute and chronic low-back pain. Cochrane Database of Systematic Reviews 3 (Art. No.: CD001824). DOI: 10.1002/14651858. CD001824.pub3.

Eubanks, JD, Lee, MJ & Cassinelli, E (2007) Prevalence of lumbar facet arthrosis and its relationship to age, sex and race: an anatomic study of cadaveric specimens. *Spine*, **32** (19), 2058–2062.

Keefe, FJ & Blumenthal, JA (1982) *Assessment strategies in behavioural medicine*. New York: Grune & Stratton.

Koes, BW, Van Tulder, MW & Ostello, R (2001) Clinical guideline for the management of low back pain in primary care – an international comparison. *Spine*, **26** (22), 2504–2514.

CHAPTER 6

Neuropathic Pain

Lesley A Colvin[1] and Suzanne Carty[2]

[1]Department of Anaesthesia, Critical Care & Pain Medicine, University of Edinburgh, Western General Hospital, Edinburgh, UK
[2]Anaesthetic Department, Musgrove Park Hospital, Taunton, UK

OVERVIEW

- Neuropathic pain is common, affecting around 6% of the population, with unique changes in the pain system that make it challenging to treat

- Diagnosis is made on a detailed history and examination. There is no specific diagnostic test and normal nerve conduction studies do *not* preclude a diagnosis of neuropathic pain. Screening tools may have a role in assisting non-specialists in diagnosis

- A range of characteristic descriptors may be used including 'shooting, stabbing or burning 'with associated 'positive'(increased) and 'negative'(decreased) sensory changes such as allodynia and hyperalgesia or numbness and reduced temperature sensation

- A range of non-standard ('adjuvant') analgesics is available: there is significant variability in response between individuals and different agents should be trialled either alone, or in combination. Standard pain killers are often ineffective

- In complex cases multidisciplinary specialist input may be required

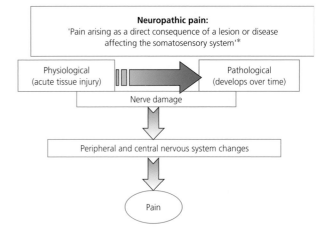

Figure 6.1 Neuropathic pain may occur as a result of changes within the peripheral or central nervous system.
*Treede, R-D, Jensen, TS, Campbell, JN, Cruccu, G, Dostrovsky, JO, Griffin, JW, et al. (2008) Neuropathic pain. Redefinition and a grading system for clinical and research purposes. *Neurology*, **70**, 1630–1635.

Table 6.1 Prevalence of neuropathic pain in the community.

Neuropathic pain disorder	Incidence per 100,000
Post-surgical pain	2000–70,000
Post-stroke (central) pain	2000–6000
Post-herpetic neuralgia (PHN)	40
Trigeminal neuralgia (TGN)	27
Complex regional pain syndrome (CRPS) type 1	26
Painful diabetic neuropathy (PDN)	15
Post-amputation pain, e.g. phantom limb pain	1

Introduction

Neuropathic pain can be initiated by, or is secondary to, an abnormality in normal sensory processing in the central or peripheral nervous system. It can be acute, for example, immediately following surgery, or may persist and become chronic (Figure 6.1). The neuropathic pain of some patients may be idiopathic in origin and, conversely, patients with clear evidence of lesions in the nervous system may have no pain at all.

Epidemiology

The exact prevalence of neuropathic pain is difficult to determine, with figures varying from 3–18% depending on the population being studied and how neuropathic pain is diagnosed (Chapter 1; Table 6.1). Neuropathic pain has been shown independently to be associated with older-age, women, unemployment and lower educational attainment. Persistent pain after surgery may continue for months or even years, with some evidence that if it is present six months after surgery, then it is likely to remain.

An awareness of when neuropathic pain may occur, a high index of suspicion when pain responds poorly to standard analgesics and asking about the characteristics of the pain may aid in identifying neuropathic pain.

Mechanisms of neuropathic pain

This is covered more fully in Chapter 2, but some of the key features are summarised in Box 6. 1.

Box 6.1 **Some of the neurobiological changes occurring in neuropathic pain**

Peripheral mechanisms
- Reduced threshold required to activate nociceptors
- Spontaneous activity in primary sensory neurons, in the absence of any peripheral stimulus
- Altered neurotransmitter production in the dorsal root ganglia

Central mechanisms
- Increased sensitivity or 'wind-up' in the spinal cord (n-methyl-d-aspartate (NMDA) receptor important role)
- Increased spontaneous background activity (balance of inhibition to excitation altered)
- Increased activity within the brainstem
- 'Central sensitisation'

Aetiology

There are many possible causes of neuropathic pain, ranging from anything causing neural compression through to specific infection with varicella zoster, as occurs in post-herpetic neuralgia (Figure 6.2). This wide range of potential aetiologies reflects the fact that neuropathic pain is not a single disease, but a spectrum of disorders that presents with specific signs and symptoms which need to be elicited in order to make a correct diagnosis.

Diagnosis

Doctors can find making the diagnosis of neuropathic pain challenging. There is no standard diagnostic procedure or test, with diagnosis

Table 6.2 Diagnosis of neuropathic pain.

	Possible	Probable	Definite
A	√	√	√
B	–		√
C	–	One of B or C	√

A = history with pain descriptors of neuropathic pain (e.g. shooting, stabbing, burning) and relevant lesion/injury of the nervous system; B = Examination showing positive (increased sensation) +/−negative (decreased sensation/numbness) sensory signs; C = additional diagnostic tests (e.g. nerve conduction studies, imaging).

Table 6.3 Screening tools for neuropathic pain.

	LANSS	DN4	NPQ	Pain DETECT	Id-Pain
Country	UK	France	USA	Germany	USA
Validated	100	160	382	392	308
Sensitivity	82–91	83	66	85	NA
Specificity	80–94	90	74	80	NA
Common symptoms	Pricking, tingling, pins and needles; electric shocks/shooting; hot/burning				
Common signs	Brush allodynia; raised pin prick threshold				

based predominantly on an accurate history and examination. Recent guidelines on the diagnosis of neuropathic pain have attempted to classify it more specifically than previously (Table 6.2).

Screening tools

Many studies have used screening tools to identify pain with neuropathic features. These do have some role in the non-specialist setting to highlight the possibility of a neuropathic type pain, but may miss 10–20% of cases. All the screening tools use a variable number of descriptors about the nature and site of the pain +/− clinical examination to define the likelihood of neuropathic pain (Table 6.3).

These screening tools include the LANSS (Leeds Assessment of Neuropathic Symptoms and Signs) or the painDETECT questionnaire, with a simplified version of the LANSS (the s-LANSS) being designed for self-completion by patients. The s-LANSS has also been validated for use in postal surveys (Box 6.2).

Box 6.2 **Summary of the s-LANSS self-report questionnaire for helping identify neuropathic pain**

- Draw on a diagram where you feel your pain
- Any pins and needles?
- Any change in skin colour of painful area?
- Is skin abnormally sensitive to touch?
- Does your pain come in bursts?
- Any burning pain?
- How does rubbing the area feel?
- How does pressing the area feel?

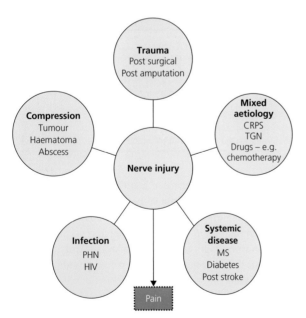

Figure 6.2 Causes of neuropathic pain. CRPS = Complex Regional Pain Syndrome; TGN = Trigeminal Neuralga; PHN = Post-Herpetic Neuralgia; HIV = Human Immunodeficiency Virus.

Features of neuropathic pain

Patients with neuropathic pain may complain of a wide range of sensory disturbance, with both increased and decreased sensation potentially occurring in the affected area. Some of the characteristics of neuropathic pain are outlined in Box 6.3.

Box 6.3 Characteristics of neuropathic pain

Spontaneous pain

- Constant burning sensation
- Intermittent shooting
- Lancinating sensations
- Electric shock-like sensations

Stimulus evoked pain

- Hyperalgesia (increased response to normally painful stimulus)
- Mechanical allodynia (pain from non-painful stimuli, e.g. light touch such as clothes brushing on the skin)
- Thermal allodynia with pain evoked by a change in temperature that is not normally painful
- 'Wind up', where a marked increase in pain is seen after repeated painful stimuli
- Secondary hyperalgesia, where the pain spreads beyond the area of the original nerve injury

---

Management of neuropathic pain

It has been shown that one of the reasons for delay in diagnosis may be lack of specific questions about the nature of the pain, which is essential in order to formulate an appropriate management plan. Patients who do not respond to basic therapies may require specialist referral.

As with any chronic pain condition, a multidisciplinary approach to management, especially for more complex cases, is important to optimise outcomes for patients.

Pharmacological treatments

There is considerable evidence for the efficacy of a range of pharmacological therapies in the management of neuropathic pain, allowing an evidence-based approach to treatment. There are several problems, however, facing clinicians in selecting the treatment that is most likely to benefit any individual.

Firstly, it is clear that the underlying mechanisms differ between patients, even those with the same syndrome. For example, in PHN some individuals may have lots of spontaneous activity in peripheral nerves maintaining their pain, whereas others may have much more central sensitisation. Using a peripherally directed treatment (e.g. a lidocaine patch) may work very well in the first case, but not at all in the second situation.

Secondly, all of the oral treatments are likely to have some form of side effect, which often precludes the necessary dose titration that is required to get an analgesic effect. This is particularly problematic in frail and elderly patients.

Thirdly, almost all available therapies require a period to reach their full analgesic effect—if a very slow dose titration is needed

Table 6.4 Treatment recommendations for peripheral neuropathic pain.

Drug	NNT
Amitriptyline	3.1
Nortryptyline	2.1
Duloxetine	4.1
Venlafaxine	4.6
Pregabalin	4.2
Gabapentin	4
Carbamazepine	2
Oxycodone	2.6
Morphine	2.5
Tramadol	3.9
Topical lidocaine patch 5%	4.4

NNT = number-needed-to treat is the number of patients who need to be treated for one to have a 50% reduction in pain (Source: Freynhagen, R & Bennett, MI (2009) Diagnosis and management of neuropathic pain. *BMJ*, **339**, 3002.)

Table 6.5 Antidepressants for neuropathic pain.

	Examples	Comments	Common adverse effects
TCAs	Amitriptyline	Dose response to 75 mg (start at 10 mg if frail); can improve sleep	Drowsiness, anticholinergic (e.g. dry mouth); *consider more selective agent (imipramine or nortriptyline if AEs troublesome)*
SNRIs	Duloxetine	Dose: 60 or 120 mg/day Most evidence for diabetic neuropathy	Nausea, somnolence constipation and reduced appetite
SSRIs	Fluoxetine	Very limited evidence (NNT ~ 15)	Nausea, insomnia

because of side effects, it may take several months to reach a potentially therapeutic dose.

There is a need to improve how a therapy is individualised to suit each patient best, and also to develop novel therapies that have fewer side effects.

There have been several reviews of the pharmacological management of neuropathic pain, with evidence for the use of anticonvulsants, antidepressants (Tricyclics or serotonin norepinephrine reuptake inhibitors (TCA or SNRIs)) or topical lidocaine as first line therapy (Table 6.4). The role of combination therapies is more difficult to assess, but in cases where there is some response to a single therapy there is a rationale for adding in other agents that act in different ways: for example, pregabalin/gabapentin and opioids, or TCAs and gabapentin.

The use of particular agents is discussed in more detail in the following sections (Table 6.5).

Anticonvulsants

The effectiveness of anticonvulsants has been established with level one evidence (good quality meta-analyses +/−systematic review) for their use in neuropathic pain. The number-needed-to-treat

(NNT) for anticonvulsants in general is around 2.5, with most of the studies having been conducted in patients with diabetic peripheral neuropathy or PHN.

Gabapentin and pregabalin are anticonvulsants commonly used in the treatment of neuropathic pain. Their mechanism of action is thought to involve presynaptic voltage-gated N-type calcium ion channels. The clinical benefits may take a few weeks to appear after titration to a therapeutic dose. The most common side effects, such as ataxia, sedation and nausea, may prevent the patient from continuing their use.

Other anticonvulsants used include carbamazepine, which acts principally on sodium channels and is particularly effective in trigeminal neuralgia. It may have significant haematological adverse effects and it is recommended that full blood counts, hepatic and renal function are monitored during use, although evidence for the value of this is limited. Newer agents include lamotrigine, which may be effective for central neuropathic pain, and topiramate.

Suggested strategy to minimise side effects
Reduce the starting dose and the size of dose increments, or increase the time between dose increments. An example for titrating pregabalin is shown in Figure 6.3.

Antidepressants

Tricyclics
There is good evidence for the use of tricyclic antidepressants (TCAs) in the management of PHN, diabetic neuropathy and other neuropathic pain. Patients may not experience clinical benefits for a few weeks with this class of drug. Moreover, they may have side

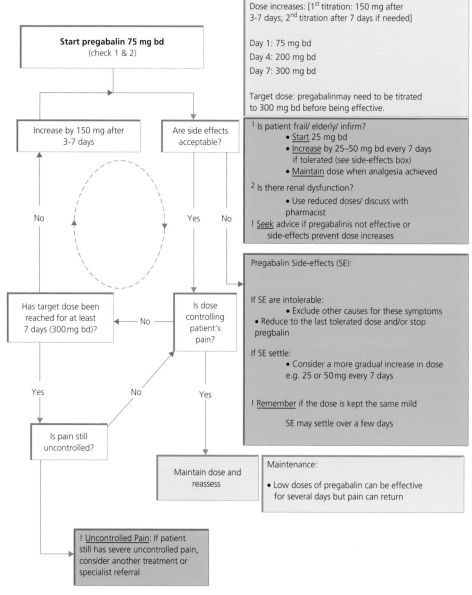

Figure 6.3 Strategy for minimising side effects when titrating pregabalin (modified from the Edinburgh Pain Assessment Tool (EPAT(C)).

effects immediately, which may reduce compliance and limit their use. TCAs can be dangerous in overdose.

Serotonin norepinephrine reuptake inhibitors (SNRIs)
More recently developed SNRIs have level one evidence for their use in neuropathic pain, with duloxetine and venlafaxine both being effective. They tend to have a better side effects profile than TCAs, although nausea may be problematic initially but often settles with time. Hypertension and ECG changes may be problematic with high doses of venlafaxine.

Selective serotonin reuptake inhibitors (SSRIs)
There is very limited evidence for the efficacy of SSRIs in the treatment of neuropathic pain.

Opioids

Opioids are increasingly recognised as an important treatment option for patients with chronic pain. They are not considered first line treatments in neuropathic pain but remain a commonly used class of drugs for this condition, with a reasonable evidence base for their use.

Although some patients will have opioid-resistant neuropathic pain, others respond well to opioids. Opioids have been shown to be most effective in intermediate-term trials, which demonstrated efficacy for spontaneous neuropathic pain. There may also be improved analgesia when used in combination with gabapentin or pregabalin. If using opioids, the use of long-acting agents is recommended, rather than immediate release preparations.

Tramadol

Tramadol has a weak action at mu opioid receptors as well as acting on the noradrenergic and serotonergic systems and there is some evidence for its use in neuropathic pain, with an NNT of 3.9.

Topical agents

One major advantage of topical agents is that they are well tolerated with minimal side effects. The topical agent with best evidence for use in neuropathic pain is the lidocaine patch (Figure 6.4). It is recommended for first line use in post-herpetic neuralgia. It has the benefit of being simple to use with minimal side effects.

Capsaicin cream 0.025% or 0.075% may also be effective for a subgroup of patients, and needs to be applied up to four times a day for maximum benefit. In practice, applying the cream frequently can be difficult for some patients and may impact on compliance.

- Cut to shape, use up to 3 patches at a time
- Effect can be cumulative – try for 4-6 weeks
- Recommended use: 12 hours out of 24 hours
  (Some patients use for longer e.g. 18 hours out of 24 with additional benefit)
- Occasional skin irritation – main side effect

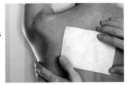

Figure 6.4 Using a lidocaine patch – practical points.

Other drugs

Ketamine is an NMDA (N-methyl-D-aspartate) receptor antagonist. When used in acute pain, it can reduce significantly the amount of opioids used in the first 24 hours post-operation. In the chronic pain setting, there is some evidence for its use in phantom limb pain, complex regional pain syndrome and post-herpetic neuralgia. No tablet preparation is currently available and side effects such as dysphoria and sedation may limit use.

Future/emerging therapies

There are a number of novel therapies that are yet to be evaluated fully in clinical practice but which may well have a useful role in the management of neuropathic pain. These include:

- *8% Capsaicin patch:* This is applied, after anaesthetising the skin for up to one hour, and may give effective pain relief for up to three months after treatment. Currently, its use is likely to be restricted to the specialist setting. Capsaicin is an agonist at the Transient Receptor Potential Vanilloid 1 (TRPV1) receptor, which is found on some subtypes of c fibres, and is involved in nociceptive processing. A one-off treatment may selectively denervate TRPV1 containing fibres.
- *Cannabinoids:* Most of the evidence to date is for multiple sclerosis-related pain, although there is some evidence from treatment-resistant peripheral neuropathic pain as well. As there are problems with limited bioavailability from oral preparations, the products being developed use the transmucosal route. Long-term follow-up studies show a relatively high incidence of minor side effects, but no development of tolerance.
- *Botulinum toxin A:* This neurotoxin has been used for some time for focal muscle spasm. It has been studied in traumatic and diabetic neuropathic pain, with some three months benefit from subcutaneous injections and little in the way of adverse effects. Further work is needed to evaluate which patients are most likely to benefit.

Stimulation techniques

Whilst having a limited evidence base, some patients will gain benefit from simple stimulation therapies such as Transcutaneous Electrical Nerve Stimulation (TENS) and acupuncture (Chapters 18 and 19).

There is some evidence for the use of the more invasive stimulation therapy: spinal cord (or dorsal column) stimulation (SCS). This requires implantation and continuing support from a specialist centre. One or more electrodes are inserted into the epidural space, either percutaneously or using an open technique. This can provide significant benefit to some patients with neuropathic pain and has been recognised as appropriate therapy for neuropathic pain by the National Institute for Health and Clinical Excellence (NICE) in the United Kingdom.

Interventions

Specific interventions such as nerve root blockade and epidurals can be useful in the diagnosis and treatment of neuropathic pain. The evidence supporting their therapeutic use is limited. These procedures are normally performed within the specialist setting. Their use is discussed further in Chapter 16.

Summary

Neuropathic pain can be a component of some chronic diseases or it can develop as a neuropathic pain disorder. Patients with neuropathic pain can experience severe symptoms, which can lead to disability and a poor quality of life. It is important to be aware of the groups of patients who are at risk and to recognise the symptoms they describe, so that their pain can be managed appropriately. A multidisciplinary and multimodal treatment approach is optimal for patients with neuropathic pain. Some treatment options are described in this chapter, including specific medications in the treatment of neuropathic pain. Above all, the selection of treatment modalities should be tailored to the individual and be based on a focused assessment of all aspects of their history and examination.

Several recent guidelines have been produced to assist in assessment and management of this challenging condition.

Further reading

Cruccu, G, Anand, P, Attal, N, Garcia-Larrea, L, Haanpaa, M, Jorum, E, *et al.* (2004) EFNS guidelines on neuropathic pain assessment. *European Journal of Neurology*, **11**, 153–162.

Freynhagen, R& Bennett, MI (2009) Diagnosis and management of neuropathic pain. *BMJ*, **339**, 3002.

Haanpaa, M, Attal, N, Backonja, M, Baron, R, Bennett, M, Bouhassira, D, *et al.* (2011) NeuPSIG guidelines on neuropathic pain assessment. *Pain*, **152**, 14–27.

http://www.medicine.ox.ac.uk/bandolier/booth/painpag/

http://www.britishpainsociety.org/pub_professional.htm

Treede, R-D, Jensen, TS, Campbell, JN, Cruccu, G, Dostrovsky, JO, Griffin, JW, *et al.* (2008) Neuropathic pain. Redefinition and a grading system for clinical and research purposes. *Neurology*, **70**, 1630–1635.

CHAPTER 7

Visceral Pain

James Maybin[1] and Michael G Serpell[2]

[1]Glasgow Royal Infirmary, Glasgow, UK
[2]University Dept of Anaesthesia, Glasgow University, Glasgow, UK

OVERVIEW

- Visceral pain is common but can be difficult to diagnose and causes considerable morbidity
- Visceral pain can initially respond to conventional analgesics
- Chronic visceral pain can be difficult to treat and may need multidisciplinary management
- Treatment of one type of visceral pain can reduce the painful symptoms from another

Introduction

The assessment and management of visceral pain are essential skills for all clinicians regardless of specialty. Visceral pain is something that everyone has experienced to some degree, but for some this can become a major disruption to everyday life. Irritable Bowel Syndrome (IBS), a dysfunctional bowel syndrome, has been estimated to account for 40–50% of all gastroenterological consultations worldwide (Figure 7.1). Dysmenorrhoea is estimated to affect 50% of menstruating women, with 10% being forced to abstain from work for a few days each month and 30% reporting no benefit from medical treatment. Myocardial ischaemia from atherosclerosis, the most frequent cause of cardiac pain, is the most common cause of death in the United States. Although common, disentangling symptoms and signs of acute visceral pathology and chronic dysfunctional pain can be a challenge for the most skilled clinician.

Pathophysiology of visceral pain

Viscera have 1% of the primary afferent innervation of somatic structures and have a much smaller cortical representation. They converge on second order neurones in the spinal cord with input from other viscera and somatic structures, which then diverge within the central nervous system (CNS). This explains the diffuse and poorly defined nature of visceral pain and also the pattern of referred pain (Table 7.1).

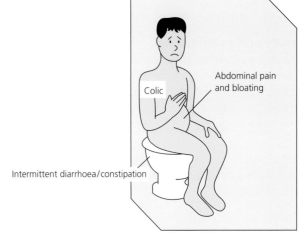

Figure 7.1 Features of Irritable Bowel Syndrome.

Table 7.1 Some of the differences and similarities between visceral and somatic pain.

	Visceral	Somatic
Character	Dull, Colicky, Diffuse	Sharp
Receptor Stimuli	Distension	Cutting, Chemical
	Ischaemia	Burns, Direct Trauma
	Inflammation	
Primary Hyperalgesia	Yes	Yes
Secondary Hyperalgesia	Yes, at referral site	Yes, around site of damage
Summation	Yes	No
Localisation	Diffuse, often referred	Precise, not referred

Adapted from McMahon, SB, Dmitrieva, N & Koltzenburg, M (1995) *British Journal of Anaesthesia*, **75**, 132–144.

The sensitivity of visceral structures varies enormously. Early surgeons, using only local anaesthesia for laparotomy, found large and small bowel insensitive to cutting, burning, crushing and tearing when applied to healthy viscera. However, viscera are sensitive to other forms of stimuli, such as distension, ischaemia and inflammation, when low intensity receptors become more responsive and previously 'silent' high threshold receptors are also recruited.

Visceral pain pathways

After nociceptor activation impulses are transmitted along slow unmyelinated C fibre tracts. There are two main types of fibre, a peptide secreting (such as substance P) and a non-peptide secreting type. It is the former type that is the most abundant and important for producing visceral hyperalgesia. These pain fibres travel alongside autonomic nerves to synapse in the dorsal horn (Figure 7.2).

The traditional view is that visceral pain transmission is carried in a few major pathways, although other pathways such as the dorsal columns, the spino (trigemino)-parabrachioamygdaloid pathway and the spinohypothalmic pathway may also be involved. As outlined in Chapter 2, peripheral and central sensitisation can develop, with a resultant increase in pain.

Visceral pain assessment

History and examination

A detailed pain history is the corner stone of every assessment (Chapter 3). For visceral pain, there are some features in particular that should be elicited during the history. The main characteristics of visceral pain are outlined in Box 7.1 and should be asked about during assessment.

> Box 7.1 **Characteristics of visceral pain.**
>
> - Intensity of pain is not linked to tissue damage
> - Diffuse and poorly localised
> - Can be colicky in nature
> - Referred to body wall
> - Classically felt in the midline (due to embryonic innervation)
> - Visceral hyperalgesia
> - Associated with autonomic symptoms and signs such as sweating, flushing and anxiety, palpitations, hypertension/hypotension

As a general rule, the intensity of discomfort bears no relationship to tissue damage. The intense pain of ureteric colic may persist well after the stone has been passed, even when there is no significant tissue damage. Conversely, some viscera are essentially insensate, for example liver, renal and lung parenchyma, and can be destroyed extensively by a neoplastic process without any pain. The innervation of the viscera is shown in Figure 7.3.

As visceral pain progresses, the pain may be referred to the somatic area that shares the second order neurone with the viscera. This is because the higher centres misinterpret the information passed to the second order neurones in the spinal cord as originating from the corresponding somatic structures (Figure 7.4).

This referred pain is better localised, can be sharper and is less likely to be associated with autonomic features, so is more like somatic pain. Further diagnostic conundrums arise when visceral referred pain is associated with hyperalgesia, the increased perception of pain to a normally painful stimulus. The hyperalgesia of referred pain is most frequently confined to the muscle but may extend superficially to the skin and so can be accompanied by

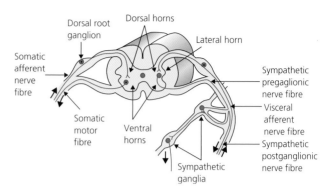

Figure 7.2 Autonomic system and dorsal.

sustained muscle contraction or sensitivity of the skin respectively (Figure 7.5).

Another consequence of central sensitisation is visceral hyperalgesia. Hyperalgesia can persist long after the initial stimulus has passed. For example, deep tenderness is often present in between menstrual cycles in the lower abdomen of women with dysmenorrhoea. Viscerovesical hyperalgesia occurs when there is amplification of pain in one viscus as the result of pathological or physiological activity in another organ that shares the same dorsal horn neurone. An example would be in women with both ureteric colic and dysmenorrhoea. These women tend to get more severe menstrual and ureteric colic pain than women with only one of the conditions. Interestingly it has been observed that treatment of one condition, for example lithotripsy for renal stones, can reduce the symptoms of another condition, for example menstrual pains.

Chronic pelvic pain in women can be difficult to diagnose as a result, but some of the common conditions and the key features are outlined in Table 7.2.

Impact of visceral pain on function

As part of the history and examination, the clinician should also focus on the effect the pain is having on the patient. Specifically, the patient should be asked about sleep pattern, effect on work, relationships with others and hobbies. Tactfully the clinician must try to establish any psychological stress, as this may be a target for intervention. Reassurance at an early stage that their pain is being taken seriously and they are not a hypochondriac (a term originally given to patients with vague abdominal pain in the upper abdomen), helps establish trust and a rapport. Both of these are essential for later management.

Visceral pain in different patient groups

The elderly often present with less severe visceral pain despite having an increased level of visceral pathology (ischaemic heart disease and intestinal obstruction). The reason for this is unclear.

There are differences between the sexes in the common types of visceral pain they present with. Females have a higher incidence of pain in the gender specific viscera, for example pelvic pain, resulting from uterine and urological (short urethra) pathology. They also have a higher incidence of gall bladder disease, whereas men have

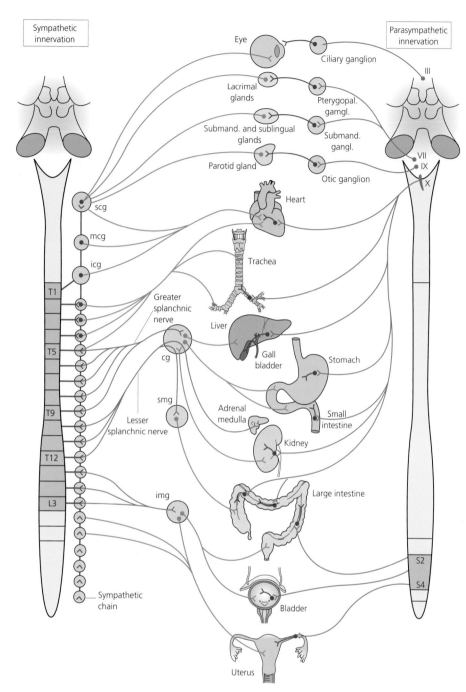

Figure 7.3 Diagram of innervation of viscera.

a higher incidence of cardiac disease (both due to lifestyle and hormonal factors). Women are also more susceptible to intestinal disease for no clear reason.

Investigations

Investigations for acute visceral pain will depend on the history and examination and are beyond the scope of this chapter. However, it is worth emphasising that the investigations themselves can perpetuate chronic visceral pain. This can be due both to physical (repeat cystocopies/colonoscopies triggering sensitisation)

and psychological mechanisms ('They cannot find what is wrong and I still have pain'). It is important, therefore, only to do investigations that are likely to contribute positively to continuing management.

Functional Magnetic Resonance Imaging (fMRI) and positron Emission Tomography have increased our understanding of the relations within the CNS and pain perception pathways.

Differences in brain activation in response to rectal distension varies between people without IBS and those who suffer from it. For example, the Anterior Cingulate Nucleus (ACN), an area

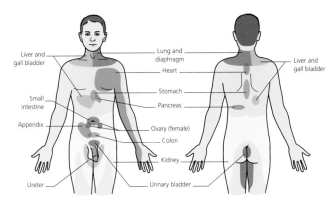

Figure 7.4 Referred pain sites.

with a high density of opioid receptors, shows increased activation in people without IBS (Figure 7.6). The ACN activation may be involved in central pain inhibition and, if bypassed, it could be a form of cerebral dysfunction associated with heightened perception of visceral pain.

Management of visceral pain

The investigation and management of visceral pain should proceed in parallel. It is obviously important to treat the cause, but pain syndromes become more severe and more resistant to treatment if they are ignored in the pursuit of a diagnosis.

The management of visceral pain can be considered in terms of three strategies:

- Pharmacological
- Psychological
- Physical intervention

The aetiology of the pain (acute pathological, chronic functional or cancer) will help to determine the best combination of therapies for the individual patient (Table 7.2).

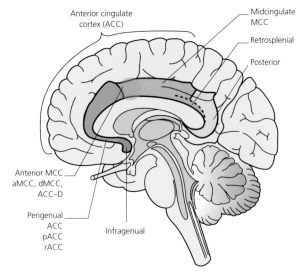

Figure 7.6 Structure of the cingulate cortex. The anterior region of the mid cingulate cortex (MCC, shown in green) is a subregion called the anterior mid cingulate cortex of the ACC (aMCC); it has a variety of other names, including the caudal ACC, the dorsal ACC (dACC), or cognitive division of the ACC (ACC-CD). pACC, anterior perigenual ACC; rACC, rostral ACC. (Reproduced with permission from Drossman, DA (2005) Brain imaging and its implications for studying centrally targeted treatments in irritable bowel syndrome: a primer for gastroemterologists. *Gut*, **54**, 569–573).

Pharmacological
Conventional analgesics

Visceral pain is a nociceptive pain and should, in the initial stages, respond to analgesics. These can be started in accordance with the WHO analgesic ladder. The use of opioid-containing analgesic for visceral pain can be effective but must be balanced against potential side effects, particularly related to the gastrointestinal tract. There are some novel approaches being used to reduce this problem, for example by combining naloxone (that stays within the GI tract) with a strong opioid. This should, in theory, reduce troublesome GI side effects, such as constipation, by blocking

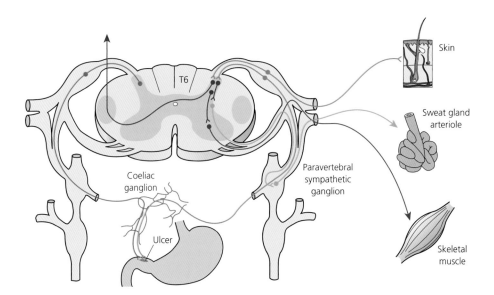

Figure 7.5 Diagram of gastric ulcer and development of hyperalgesia.

Table 7.2 Common causes of pelvic pain.

Organ System	Pathological Process	Key for Diagnosis	Treatment options
Gynaecological	Endometriosis	Laparoscopy	Medical: hormone therapy Surgical: ablation, hysterectomy and bilateral salpingo-oophorectomy, ablation of uterine nerves
	Pelvic Venous congestion	Laparoscopy/ultrasound/Venography	Medical: gonadotrophin analogues, progestogens Surgical: hysterectomy and salpingo-oophorectomy
	Vulvodynia Essential (Diagnosis of exclusion)	Dysaesthesia and hypersensitivity to mechanical stimuli	Antineuropathic medication CBT Simple analgesia
	Vulvar dermatoses Vulvar vestubulitis	History, examination +/−biopsy and microbiology	Antivirals, antifungals, hygiene advice
Urinary Tract	Acute/Chronic urinary tract infection	Urine microscopy and culture	Antimicrobial therapy
	Urethral syndrome	Symptoms of lower urinary tract irritation but no cause found	Modification of voiding habits, urethral dilatation, urethrotomy, improvement of pelvic floor muscles
	Interstitial cystitis (chronic inflammation of the bladder)	Cystoscopy and biopsy	Modification of voiding habits, bladder distension, TCA
Gastrointestinal	IBS	History with absence of abnormal findings on investigation	CBT Simple analgesia Anticholinergics
	Adhesions	Laparoscopy	Surgical division
Musculoskeletal	Nerve Entrapement		
	Ilioinguinal – stabbing pain in groin, labia and inner thigh, exacerbated by exercise *Abdominal Cutaneous*- stabbing or prickling pain exacerbated with coughing or straining abdominal muscles	History and examination	Nerve block with local anaesthetic and steroid. Neurolytic procedures such as cryotherapy, radiofrequency ablation or injection of phenol are rarely done for non-malignant pain due to the risk of chronic deafferentation pain.
	Muscular Trigger Points	History and examination	Injection of LA and steroid, TENS, acupuncture
Psychological	Anxiety/depression	Absence of other findings on investigation. Presence of other psychological morbidity	Multidisciplinary approach. Pain Management Programmes.

CBT: cognitive behavioural therapy; TENS: transcutaneous electrical nerve stimulation; TCA: tricyclic antidepressants; LA: local anaesthetic; IBS: irritable bowel syndrome

peripheral opioid receptors, but without loss of centrally mediated analgesia (Figure 7.7).

Organ specific drugs

Nitrates and beta blockers are often used for angina. Other examples include anticholinergics for intestinal spasm in IBS, proton pump inhibitors for dyspepsia and hormonal treatments for endometriosis and dysmenorrhoea.

Adjuvants

Given that in chronic visceral pain syndromes there are likely to be changes in pain processing, with sensitisation at different levels, there is a rationale for using agents that will target this sensitisation. Low dose tricyclic antidepressants, such as amitriptyline, can help to control symptoms in IBS and has been used with success in both adult and paediatric patient groups. Gabapentin, sodium channel blockers and ketamine have also all been used with varying success.

Psychological

Psychological input is an important component in managing all chronic pain conditions. Initially this may include patient education and cognitive behavioural therapies such as stress management, relaxation and diversion strategies. For more complex cases, specialist input from a multidisciplinary team to address pain management may be required.

Physical intervention

Simple physical therapies include acupuncture, transcutaneous electrical nerve stimulation (TENS) and physiotherapy (Chapters

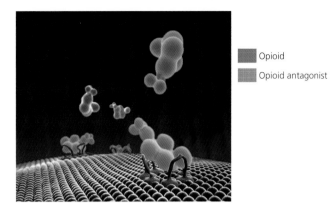

Opioid

Opioid antagonist

Figure 7.7 Opioid antagonists can prevent gastrointestinal binding of strong opioids and thus reduce side effects, such as constipation. This relies on antagonists such as naloxone having a greater affinity for opioid receptors in the gut than the agonist. (Reproduced with permission from Napp Pharmaceuticals).

17–19). Side effects are minimal and these treatments should always be considered before more invasive techniques. Complex interventional methods are reserved for pain that has a defined anatomical lesion causing it or when all other methods have failed to control the pain, as they have considerable risks and side effects. These include nerve plexus blocks, for example coeliac plexus for pancreatic cancer pain, intrathecal drug delivery systems, spinal cord and deep brain stimulation (Figure 7.6; Chapter 16).

Summary

Visceral pain is a common complaint and can cause significant morbidity and mortality. A detailed history and examination are essential foundations for effective management of patients with visceral pain. Management should always proceed in parallel with continuing investigations to reduce unnecessary delays in treatment. Through research, new pain pathways and cellular mechanisms are being discovered which may improve the success for pharmacological and physical intervention. In combination with psychological therapies these form the basics of a modern, multidisciplinary approach to the management of patients with visceral pain.

Further reading

Aitkenhead, AR, Rowbotham, DJ (Smith, G (2001) *Textbook of Anaesthesia*, 4th edn. Churchill Livingstone Publishing.

Carr, DB (Editor-in-chief) (2005) *Visceral Pain. Pain Clinical Updates*, Volume XIII, No. 6. International Association for the Study of Pain.

Cervero, F & Laird, JMA (1999) Visceral Pain. *Lancet*, **353**, 2145–2148

Drossman, DA (2005) Brain imaging and its implications for studying centrally targeted treatments in irritable bowel syndrome: a primer for gastroemterologists. *Gut*, **54**, 569–573.

Lynch, ME & Campbell, F (2008) A systematic review of the effect of waiting for treatment for chronic pain. *Pain*, **136**, 97–116.

McMahon, SB, Dmitrieva, N & Koltzenburg, M (1995) *British Journal of Anaesthesia*, **75**, 132–144.

CHAPTER 8

Post-surgical Pain

Susan Nimmo and Lesley Dickson

Department of Anaesthetics, Critical Care and Pain Medicine, Western General Hospital, Edinburgh, UK

OVERVIEW

- Chronic pain following surgery is a common and increasingly recognised problem

- Severe and poorly controlled acute pain is one of the most consistent risk factors for the development of chronic post-surgical pain; this may include the development of acute neuropathic pain

- Diagnosis of post-operative neuropathic pain is a clinical one based on a careful history of the pain

- Effective control of post-operative nociceptive and neuropathic pain where identified, is currently our best strategy aimed at reducing chronic post-operative pain, although the efficacy of this approach is unproven at present

- Post-operative neuropathic pain is poorly responsive to opioids and usually requires treatment with specific antineuropathic medication.

Introduction

For the majority of patients, pain following surgery, while unpleasant, is usually a time limited event which should be well controlled with multimodal analgesia and ends with complete resolution of the pain (Figure 8.1) It is increasingly recognised, however, that a small proportion of patients continue to have significant levels of pain related to a surgical intervention beyond the anticipated time for resolution and that a number of these will develop chronic pain following surgery. As the duration of hospital stay after surgery is shortened, it is essential to ensure that acute post-surgical pain is managed optimally both in the inpatient and community settings.

This leads to two issues:

- What changes, if any, need to be made to standard post-operative multimodal analgesia to control prolonged post-operative pain?
- Is it possible to reduce the incidence of chronic pain related to surgery?

ABC of Pain, First edition. Edited by Lesley A Colvin and Marie Fallon.
© 2012 Blackwell Publishing Ltd. Published 2012 by Blackwell Publishing Ltd.

Assessment

There are four main groups of patients which have prolonged pain following surgery. Diagnosis of the problem and institution of appropriate management depends on taking a careful pain history and examination (Box 8.1). Failure to ask questions about the site and character of the pain make accurate diagnosis much harder. Some additional tools are also available if appropriate to the situation; these include neuropathic pain questionnaires such as the self-report Leeds Assessment of Neuropathic Symptoms and Signs (s-LANSS) (Chapter 6).

Box 8.1 Taking a pain history

- Patients own verbal report of pain (where possible)
- Circumstances associated with onset of pain
- Pain intensity at rest and on movement (using pain assessment tool)
- Character (intermittent or constant)
- Location and radiation
- Exacerbating and relieving factors
- Effect of pain on other activities including sleep
- Current medications and other treatments for pain
- Associated symptoms (e.g. nausea)
- Previous or coexisting pain/medical conditions
- Vital signs – respiratory rate, pulse, blood pressure, SpO2
- Behavioural signs (facial expressions, crying, restlessness, guarding or rubbing of the affected area)

Aetiology of prolonged pain following surgery

Surgical causes

The duration of pain following surgery will be protracted if surgical complications arise, such as a wound infection, where pain will remain in the surgical area. Alternatively, a patient may develop new pain resulting from a post-operative complication, for example pleuritic chest pain associated with a post-operative chest infection. It is important to take a history from the patient and undertake a thorough clinical assessment in order to diagnose these problems, since specific management is likely to be necessary and should resolve the problem. Continued multimodal analgesia is likely to be effective in controlling these types of pain.

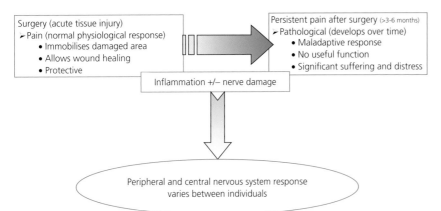

Figure 8.1 Surgical tissue injury normally heals with resolution of pain within days to weeks.

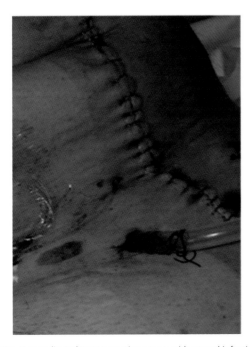

Figure 8.2 A complicated post-operative course with wound infection may predispose to persistent pain.

It has been shown, however, that prolonged wound pain due to infection or haematoma is one of the risk factors for development of chronic postoperative pain (Figure 8.2).

Prior pain sensitisation

The pain pathway is a dynamic entity which not only provides pain signalling to the central nervous system but also undergoes a series of changes known as peripheral and central sensitisation in response to a continuing pain stimulus (Chapter 2). For the majority of individuals and/or pain episodes these changes would appear to be reversible. However, it is recognised clinically that there are some patients who appear to retain a 'hyped up' pain pathway and, while not suffering from chronic pain, do suffer from more severe and more protracted pain than might be anticipated. Again most of these patients respond well to multimodal analgesia but it may be necessary to use higher dosing schedules and slow the pace of step down analgesia.

Analgesic tolerance

Patients who present for surgery who are already taking opioid medication, either therapeutically or off prescription, will have developed a degree of tolerance to opioids which makes effective post-operative pain management more difficult, particularly if an opioid-based technique such as patient-controlled analgesia is used. Again, these patients require a higher dose of opioids to be given and will usually take longer to step down their analgesia. It is also likely that at least some of these patients will have preceding pain sensitisation in addition to having tolerance. There is some evidence, for example, that patients on methadone maintenance for substance misuse may have lower pain thresholds.

Development of neuropathic pain

Taking a full pain history (symptoms suggesting neuropathic pain are outlined in Box 8.2) or using a neuropathic pain questionnaire, such as the s-LANSS, demonstrates that up to 10% of patients develop symptoms compatible with neuropathic pain post-operatively. A neuropathic component to the overall post-operative pain should probably also be considered if a patient has persistent poor pain control in the face of adequate levels of multimodal analgesia.

> **Box 8.2 Symptoms suggesting the development of neuropathic pain**
>
> - Pain in the absence of ongoing tissue damage
> - Pain in an area of sensory loss
> - Paroxysmal or spontaneous pain
> - Allodynia (pain in response to non-painful stimuli)
> - Hyperalgesia (increased pain in response to painful stimuli)
> - Dysaesthesia
> - Characteristic of pain different from nociception (e.g. burning, stabbing)
> - Poor response to opioids or increased opioid use
> - Presence of major neurological deficit (e.g. brachial plexus injury)

Neuropathic pain is pain that is generated within the pain pathway either peripherally or centrally (or both) as a result of damage to the pathway as a consequence of surgery (Chapter 6). While a direct cause and effect is hard to prove, it is considered

Table 8.1 Estimated incidence of chronic pain following surgery.

Operation	Incidence of pain > 3 months duration (%)
Amputation	50–85
Thoracotomy	5–65
Mastectomy	20–50
Cholecystectomy: open	7–48
Cholecystectomy: laparoscopic	3–56
Hernia repair	6–30
Hip replacement	12
Caesarian section	6

likely that development of neuropathic symptoms in the immediate post-operative period is a precursor to chronic post-operative pain.

The role of surgery in the generation of chronic pain conditions is becoming increasingly recognised and accepted. The incidence varies following different surgical procedures but is remarkably high in some series (Table 8.1). Chronic pain following surgery can have a detrimental effect on quality of life and lead to disabling limitations to an individual's activities.

Risk factors for the development of chronic pain following surgery

A variety of studies and systematic reviews have attempted to identify risk factors for the development of chronic pain following surgery in the hope of improving understanding of this condition (Box 8.3). This could then lead to strategies for improved management of patients and, more importantly, preventative measures.

Box 8.3 **Risk factors for the development of chronic pain following surgery**

- Direct nerve damage by surgery or trauma
- Severe and poorly controlled acute pain
- Pre-existing chronic pain
- Repeated surgical procedures
- Fear, catastrophizing and poor post-operative recovery of function
- Previous severe uncontrolled acute pain
- Pre-operative opioid use

Given the large variation in the occurrence of chronic pain for individual operations it seems likely that its aetiology is both multifactorial and complex. Chronic post-operative pain usually has a neuropathic component, suggesting that either peripheral or more central pain pathway damage may be involved. Certainly, direct nerve damage could be invoked in amputation pain or thoracotomy pain for example. However, not all patients with demonstrable nerve lesions following surgery develop pain, and pain can occur following nerve sparing surgery. The extent of surgery may be a factor in some cases; for example, laparoscopic hernia surgery has a lower incidence of pain than open procedures in some series. However, again, this is not a consistent factor. There is also the possibility that an individual's genetic makeup may alter their risk of developing chronic pain, with some emerging evidence for this (See 'Further reading', Tegeder et al.).

Severe and poorly controlled acute pain is one of the more consistent risk factors identified for development of chronic pain (Figure 8.3). It is not known, however, whether this identifies a patient with a likelihood of severe pain in any modality or if severe acute pain is a causative factor. Certainly, severe acute pain could result in the type of peripheral and central sensitisation events described above, which might lead to chronic pain. Conversely, there is little evidence that good post-operative pain control reduces the incidence of chronic pain. However, if central sensitisation is invoked as a mechanism, then most of our multimodal acute pain management would not be adequate throughout the post-operative period to avoid sensitisation completely, which goes some way to explaining the lack of benefit.

Fear, catastrophising and poor post-operative recovery of function and quality of life are all factors that have been found to be associated with chronic post-operative pain.

Other chronic pain modalities, such as the presence of fibromyalgia, painful Raynaud's phenomenon, migraine and irritable bowel syndrome, are recognised as risk factors for chronic post-surgical pain and patients with these conditions should have this taken into consideration when making decisions about surgery and their post-operative analgesia.

Can post-operative neuropathic pain be prevented or reduced?

Given that chronic pain following surgery often has a neuropathic element which is harder to treat than nociceptive pain, strategies

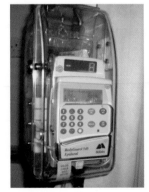
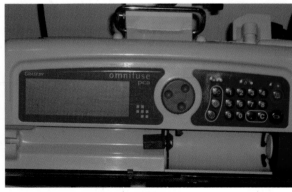

Figure 8.3 Local anaesthetic techniques and potent opioids are the mainstays of acute post-operative pain management: (a) epidural infusion device; (b) patient controlled analgesia pump.

(a)

(b)

Table 8.2 Suggested initial and maintenance doses of oral antineuropathic pain agents used in acute neuropathic pain, and the side effects most commonly seen in this context. The British National Formulary (BNF) should be consulted for more detailed information on these agents.

	Dose: Initial	Dose : Maintenance	Commonly seen side effects
Gabapentin	100–300 mg determined by age and frailty	600 mg three times daily	Sedation Muscle twitching
Pregabalin	25–75 mg determined by age and frailty	Up to 600 mg daily divided into two or three doses	Sedation
Carbamazepine	100 mg twice daily	200 mg four times daily	Rare risk of haematological disorders, Stevens Johnson syndrome and liver dysfunction
Amitriptyline	10 mg	75 mg	Sedation, dry mouth, postural hypotension, dysphoria

to avoid the development of chronic pain post surgery are being sought. At present, preventative strategies are limited to avoiding unnecessary surgery, particularly for individuals considered to be high risk for developing chronic post-operative pain, and the optimal provision of multimodal analgesia for those patients who do have surgery. Whilst there is evidence suggestive of benefit if some of the antineuropathic pain agents listed in Table 8.2 are given perioperatively, this is not yet of proven advantage and the side effects of many of these agents preclude their routine use in all patients. There is some limited evidence that a single dose of gabapentin (up to 500 mg) may be useful in the acute setting, although the impact of this on chronic pain is not clear.

Currently, clinical management is aimed at providing the best possible perioperative analgesia, recognising that poorly controlled post-operative pain is one of the more consistent risk factors for chronic post-surgical pain, and also at prompt recognition and management of post-operative neuropathic pain.

Optimal multimodal analgesia should be achieved and continued for the duration of post-operative pain (Figure 8.4). The use of local anaesthetic techniques, where appropriate and possible, would seem to be of benefit, since successful local anaesthesia is the only pain treatment modality which can achieve zero pain on movement. However, again there is limited evidence at present that the use of these techniques reduces the incidence of chronic post-operative pain.

How is post-operative neuropathic pain managed?

The importance of careful assessment and reassessment after treatment cannot be over-emphasised. This can be particularly challenging when patients are rapidly discharged after surgery, and may involve patients/carers being provided with appropriate information and support in the community. If acute neuropathic symptoms develop then consideration should be given to converting the patient to an opioid which has some evidence of benefit in neuropathic pain, such as oxycodone or tramadol.

There are a number of agents with known antineuropathic activity that can be titrated to improve or resolve neuropathic symptoms in the acute situation: expert advice from local pain teams may need to be sought (Table 8.2).

Possible treatment options

Ketamine is an n-methyl-d -aspartate (NMDA) receptor antagonist. The NMDA receptor plays a key role in central sensitisation (Chapters 2 and 6). Ketamine therefore has good analgesic activity and can also be effective in the control of acute neuropathic symptoms. It can be given by a variety of routes but is most commonly prescribed as an intravenous or subcutaneous infusion for acute neuropathic pain. Improvement in symptoms would be anticipated

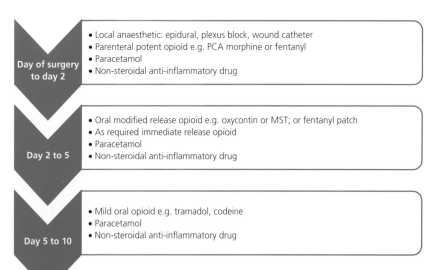

Day of surgery to day 2
- Local anaesthetic: epidural, plexus block, wound catheter
- Parenteral potent opioid e.g. PCA morphine or fentanyl
- Paracetamol
- Non-steroidal anti-inflammatory drug

Day 2 to 5
- Oral modified release opioid e.g. oxycontin or MST; or fentanyl patch
- As required immediate release opioid
- Paracetamol
- Non-steroidal anti-inflammatory drug

Day 5 to 10
- Mild oral opioid e.g. tramadol, codeine
- Paracetamol
- Non-steroidal anti-inflammatory drug

Figure 8.4 Optimal multimodal analgesia. The analgesic choices at each step will vary dependent on operative severity, side effects and contra-indications to individual agents. Similarly the timing of step-down of analgesia must be tailored to individual patient requirements both in terms of analgesics prescribed and timing of step-down.

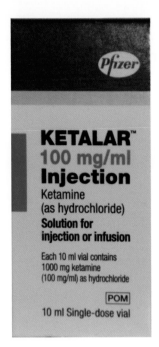

Figure 8.5 Ketamine can be highly effective as an antineuropathic agent in the acute setting. Currently no tablet formulation is available for chronic use.

fairly quickly, within a few hours of commencing the infusion. Doses of between 5 and 15 mg per hour are used, and provided the lowest effective rate is used, side effects are minimised. Patients should however, be warned that they may experience nightmares and hallucinations which are often unpleasant. A low dose of oral haloperidol (2 mg) may be helpful for this. If the symptoms are intolerable then ketamine will have to be discontinued and alternatives sought. It is also possible to control these symptoms with benzodiazepines, but in combination with other sedative agents, such as opioids and ketamine, this is likely to make patients unacceptably drowsy and as a result is not used routinely in this situation (Figure 8.5).

Local anaesthetics act by reducing sodium channel activity and, hence, can be effective in neuropathic pain treatment, where there may be alterations in the sodium channel activity in damaged nerves. Infusions of the commonly used local anaesthetic, lidocaine, either subcutaneously or intravenously, may be tried but must be done with appropriate monitoring and trained staff in case of toxicity, which can include seizures and cardiac arrhythmias.

Clinical experience shows that other antineuropathic agents, such as the antiepileptics, gabapentin and pregabalin, and carbamazepine or tricyclic antidepressants, such as amitriptyline, may be effective for some patients with acute neuropathic pain. However, neither the optimal agent in this situation nor the efficacy of agents in terms

of reducing chronic as opposed to acute symptoms is yet known. Further research is required in these areas.

Summary

Chronic pain following surgery may be associated with poorly controlled post-operative pain, which may be simply a failure of effective analgesia or may be associated with the early generation of neuropathic pain. There is an increased risk if surgical complications have occurred, possibly due to more protracted generation of pain and increased potential for neurological damage and resultant neuropathic pain.

It is hoped that continued improvements in acute post-operative pain management will help control the generation of chronic pain, as should early targeted intervention for neuropathic pain symptoms.

If risk factors for chronic pain are understood better then patients at risk may be identified pre-operatively. This might allow tailoring of surgery, for example the use of a laparoscopic procedures with reduced tissue trauma or even avoidance of non-essential operations altogether. If surgery proceeds then pain relief could be tailored specifically for that individual, with the use of regional block techniques, which would be most effective in reducing pain, and also early use of antineuropathic treatments.

The recognition that surgery is a significant contributor to the incidence of chronic pain has been slow. It is to be hoped that with improved recognition and assessment of the occurrence of chronic postoperative pain, coupled with advances in understanding the pathophysiology within the pain pathway, that advances will be made in the future which allow more effective treatments and, ultimately, prevention of chronic pain following surgery.

Further reading

Crombie, IK, Davies, HTO & Macrae, WA (1998) Cut and thrust: antecedent surgery and trauma among patients attending a chronic pain clinic. *Pain*, **76**, 167–171.

Kehlet, H, Jensen, TS & Woolf, CJ (2006) Persistent postsurgical pain: risk factors and prevention. *Lancet*, **367**, 1618–1625.

Macrae, WA (2008) Chronic post-surgical pain: 10 years on. *British Journal of Anaesthesia*, **101**, 77–86.

Straube, S, Derry, S, Moore, RA, Wiffen, PJ & McQuay, HJ (2010) Single dose oral gabapentin for established acute postoperative pain in adults. *Cochrane Database of Systematic Reviews* 5 (Art. No.: CD008183). doi: 10.1002/14651858.CD008183.pub2.

Tegeder, M, Costigan, RS, Griffin, A, *et al.* (2006) GTP cyclohydrolase and tetrahydrobiopterin regulate pain sensitivity and persistence. *Nature Medicine*, **12**, 1269–1277.

Wilson, JA, Colvin, LA & Power, I (2002) Acute neuropathic pain after surgery. *Bulletin 15, The Royal College of Anaesthetists*, 739–743.

CHAPTER 9

Headache and Orofacial Pain

Anne MacGregor[1] and Joanna M Zakrzewska[2]

[1] St Bartholomew's and the London School of Medicine and Dentistry, London, UK
[2] Consultant in Oral Medicine, University College London Hospitals NHS Foundation Trust, London, UK

OVERVIEW

- Headache and orofacial pain are common disorders presenting to all healthcare professionals
- Primary headaches are independent diseases with specific management strategies
- Secondary headaches and orofacial pains are treated by management of the underlying conditions
- Accurate diagnosis is essential in order for the most appropriate management strategies to be employed
- Investigations are indicated only if a secondary cause is suspected

---

Introduction

Headache and orofacial disorders comprise a heterogenous group of disorders of varying prevalence (Box 9.1). Despite being extremely common, headache and orofacial disorders are under-recognised and under-diagnosed and can result in considerable pain and disability. The second edition of the International Classification of Headache Disorders (ICHD-II) lists more than100 headache and facial pain conditions (see Further reading). These can be further classified by cause (Figure 9.1). In this chapter, strategies for diagnosis are outlined and headache and facial pain that is often misdiagnosed or inadequately managed by non-specialists is the focus.

Box 9.1 Causes of headache and facial pain

Prevalence >10%
Hangover
Tension-type headache
Fever
Metabolic disorders
Sinusitis
Migraine
Temporomandibular disorders
Persistent idiopathic facial pain

Prevalence >1% ≤10%
Medication overuse headache
Idiopathic stabbing headache

Prevalence ≤1%
Giant cell arteritis
Cranial neuralgias

Trigeminal
Glossopharyngeal
Occipital

Trigeminal autonomic cephalalgias (TACs)

Cluster headache
Chronic Paroxysmal hemicrania
Short-lasting unilateral neuralgiform headache attacks with conjunctival injection and tearing (SUNCT), Short-lasting unilateral neuralgiform headache attacks with autonomic features (SUNA)

Trigeminal neuropathy
Post-herpetic neuralgia

History

The history is a crucial step in diagnosis (Box 9.2). Patients often present with more than one type of pain, so a separate history is required for each. In the emergency setting, there may not be time to take a full history. The first task is to exclude conditions requiring more urgent intervention by eliciting any warning features (Table 9.1).

Box 9.2 Approach to the history

1 **How many different headache types does the patient experience?**
Separate histories are necessary for each. It is reasonable to concentrate on the most bothersome to the patient but others should always attract some enquiry in case they are clinically important.

2 **Time questions**
a. Why consulting now?
b. How recent in onset?
c. How frequent, and what temporal pattern (especially distinguishing between episodic and daily or unremitting)?
d. How long lasting?

ABC of Pain, First edition. Edited by Lesley A Colvin and Marie Fallon.
© 2012 Blackwell Publishing Ltd. Published 2012 by Blackwell Publishing Ltd.

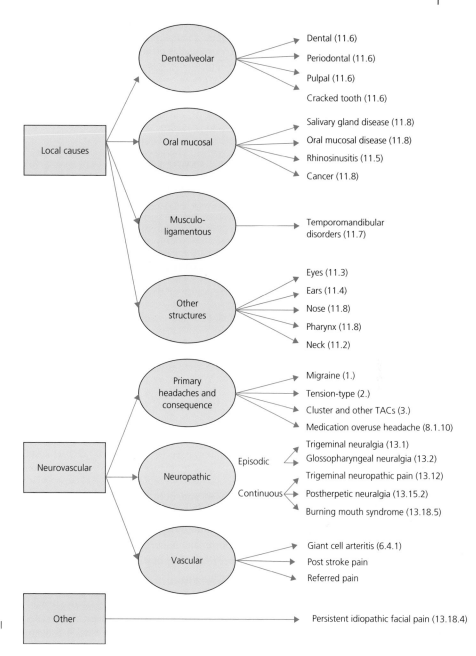

Dentoalveolar
  → Dental (11.6)
  → Periodontal (11.6)
  → Pulpal (11.6)
  → Cracked tooth (11.6)

Oral mucosal
  → Salivary gland disease (11.8)
  → Oral mucosal disease (11.8)
  → Rhinosinusitis (11.5)
  → Cancer (11.8)

Musculo-ligamentous
  → Temporomandibular disorders (11.7)

Other structures
  → Eyes (11.3)
  → Ears (11.4)
  → Nose (11.8)
  → Pharynx (11.8)
  → Neck (11.2)

Local causes

Primary headaches and consequence
  → Migraine (1.)
  → Tension-type (2.)
  → Cluster and other TACs (3.)
  → Medication overuse headache (8.1.10)

Neuropathic
  Episodic
    → Trigeminal neuralgia (13.1)
    → Glossopharyngeal neuralgia (13.2)
  Continuous
    → Trigeminal neuropathic pain (13.12)
    → Postherpetic neuralgia (13.15.2)
    → Burning mouth syndrome (13.18.5)

Neurovascular

Vascular
  → Giant cell arteritis (6.4.1)
  → Post stroke pain
  → Referred pain

Other
  → Persistent idiopathic facial pain (13.18.4)

Figure 9.1 Classification of headache and orofacial pain (ICHD-II code). TACs: trigeminal autonomic cephalalgias.

3 Character questions
  a. Intensity of pain
  b. Nature and quality of pain
  c. Site and spread of pain
  d. Associated symptoms
4 Cause questions
  a. Predisposing and/or trigger factors
  b. Aggravating and/or relieving factors
  c. Family history of similar headache
5 Response to headache questions
  a. What does the patient do during the headache?
  b. How much is activity (function) limited or prevented?
  c. What medication has been and is used, and in what manner?

6 State of health between attacks
  a. Completely well, or residual or persisting symptoms?
  b. Concerns, anxieties, fears about recurrent attacks, and/or their cause

Based on: MacGregor, EA, Steiner, TJ & Davies, PTG (2010) Guidelines for All Healthcare Professionals in the Diagnosis and Management of Migraine, Tension-Type, Cluster and Medication-Overuse Headache. Available at: http://www.bash.org.uk.

Examination

The examination will reflect the suspected diagnosis, particularly in the case of local disease of the oral cavity. A good light and expertise

Table 9.1 Warning features in the history.

Symptoms	Possible diagnosis	Investigation
Thunderclap headache (intense headache with abrupt or 'explosive' onset)	Subarachnoid haemorrhage	CT without contrast LP (if CT normal or unavailable)
Headache with atypical aura (duration >1 hour, or including motor weakness)	TIA Ischaemic stroke	CT with contrast/MRI
Fever	Meningitis	LP Blood cultures
History of HIV or syphilis	Encephalopathy	Antibody testing LP MRI
History of cancer	Secondary brain metastases	CT with contrast/MRI
New onset headache over age 50	Giant cell arteritis	ESR/CRP Temporal artery biopsy
	Glaucoma	Ophthalmological review
Progressive headache worsening over weeks or months Symptoms of raised intracranial pressure • Drowsiness • Postural related headache • Vomiting New onset seizures Cognitive or personality changes Progressive neurological deficit • Weakness • Sensory loss • Dysphasia • Ataxia	Intracranial space-occupying lesion	CT with contrast/MRI
Progressive sensory loss over the face and/or intraorally	Intracranial space-occupying lesion	Neurophysiological testing, CT or MRI

CT: computed tomography; CRP: C-reactive protein; ESR: erythrocyte sedimentation rate; LP: lumbar puncture; MRI: magnetic resonance imaging; TIA: transient ischaemic attack

in examining the oral tissues is necessary. The head and neck should be carefully examined. Assess tenderness over the temporal arteries as well tenderness in the scalp, neck muscles and muscles of mastication. Examination of patients with temporomandibular disorders (TMD) involves the application of pressure to a variety of specific anatomical sites to see if they are tender (trigger points). The range of movements of the mandible is then evaluated in vertical opening, protrusive and lateral positions. A brief but thorough neurological examination, especially of the cranial nerves, should be undertaken, particularly if the diagnosis is uncertain or intracranial pathology is suspected. Fundoscopy is mandatory in all patients presenting with headache. Examination of the cranial nerves is particularly important for orofacial pain. General examination is indicated if headaches are considered secondary to systemic disease.

Investigations

There is no indication for investigations of primary headaches and they should be undertaken only if a secondary headache is suspected. If autoimmune disorders are suspected then blood tests may be indicated. Non-contrast computed tomography (CT) with axial and coronal sections is indicated for sinusitis, rhinogenic causes of pain or if malignancy is suspected. Magnetic resonance imaging (MRI) is useful to evaluate internal derangement in TMD. MRI and/or magnetic resonance angiography (MRA) can evaluate

intracranial pathology. Special thin cut MRIs of the posterior fossa are needed to identify trigeminal nerve root compressions.

Management issues

Patients' beliefs are fundamental and must be clarified before treatment is initiated (Box 9.3). Severity of disease, impact on quality of life, insight and chronicity will impact on adherence to treatment as well as how the family views the condition (Box 9.4). The approach must, therefore, be a biopsychosocial one.

Box 9.3 **Questions to ask patients about their expectations for management**

- What are the most important results you hope to receive from this treatment?
- Are you expecting a complete cure or just relief of pain?
- How much reduction in suffering would be acceptable if complete reduction were not possible?
- Are you looking for rapid results or are you prepared to accept slow change?
- How important is your quality of life and how much can this be compromised to achieve better pain control?
- What help do you need to develop active coping skills?

Source: Zakrzewska, JM (2002) Facial pain: neurological and non-neurological. *J Neurol Neurosurg Psychiat*, **72** (suppl II), ii27–ii32. Reproduced with permission of BMJ Publishing.

Box 9.4 **Aims of management**

- Eliminate or minimise headache and orofacial pain
- Eliminate or minimise negative cognitive, behavioural and emotional factors
- Increase efficacy of drug therapy by careful choice
- Improve adherence by ensuring that the patient is well informed
- Encourage self-management which increases control over pain.

Source: Zakrzewska, JM (2002) Facial pain: neurological and non-neurological. *J Neurol Neurosurg Psychiat*, **72** (suppl II), ii27–ii32. Reproduced with permission of BMJ Publishing.

A daily record of symptoms, trigger factors and treatments taken is an invaluable aid to diagnosis and management, particularly if more than one condition is present (Figure 9.2). Review of diary cards can also identify what medication is taken and if it is taken in adequate doses at the optimal time. Symptom diaries can help identify triggering factors which can then be modified. Patients should be made aware of the effects that chronic pain can have on mood and health. Providing patients with a jargon free holistic explanation for their pain, highlighting that all pain is processed in the brain can help many patients to an improved understanding and to appreciate the challenges of living with chronic pain. Patient support groups for a variety of these conditions exist and can provide patients with further information and contact with fellow sufferers. This type of 'information prescription' can be of more value than medication in helping patients come to terms with their disorder and in learning to develop coping strategies.

Primary headaches

The diagnosis of primary headache is based on the history and the absence of physical signs. For more detailed information on management, see The British Association for the Study of Headache (BASH) guidelines.

the City of London Migraine Clinic
22 Charterhouse Square · London EC1M 6DX · Tel: 020 7251 3322 · Fax: 020 7490 2183 · Website: www.migraineclinic.org.uk

Month __June__ Year__2007__ Other Drugs: Daily Preventative: Name__None__ .... Dose ....
Name. __O. V. Dose__ DOB__11/11/1950__ Hormonal treatments: Name__None__

Date	Day	Headache or Migraine	Severity	Time Started	Nausea	Vomiting	What treatment did you take	Time taken
1	MON	H	mod	5.10am	no	no	analgesic	5.10am
2	TUE	H	mod	5.00am	no	no	analgesic	5.00am
3	WED	H	mod	5.00am	no	no	analgesic	5.00am
4	THU	H	mod	5.30am	no	no	analgesic	5.30am
5	FRI	migraine	severe	6.00am	yes	no	triptan	6.00am
6	SAT	H	mod	6.10am	yes	no	triptan	6.10am
7	SUN	-	-	-	-	-	-	-
8	MON	migraine	severe	4.30am	yes	yes	triptan	7am/3pm
9	TUE	migraine	severe	4.30am	yes	no	triptan	4.30am
10	WED	migraine	severe	3.00am	yee	no	triptan	3am/7am
11	THU	H	mod	7.00am	no	no	analgesic	7.00am
12	FRI	H	mod	12.10am	no	no	analgesic	12.10am
13	SAT	H	mod	7.00am	no	no	analgesic	7.00am
14	SUN	H	mod	7.30am	no	no	analgesic	7.30am
15	MON	H	mod	7.10am	no	no	analgesic	7.10am

Figure 9.2 Diary card showing migraine on the background of daily headache. Given the use of symptomatic treatment on more than two days a week, medication overuse headache is probable.

Table 9.2 Characteristics of migraine.

Prevalence	1 in 6
Male:female ratio	1:3
Age group most affected	30–50 years
Frequency of attacks	Episodic
Duration of attacks	4–72 hours
Intensity of pain	Moderate or severe
Quality of pain	Deep, pulsating
Site of pain	Often unilateral but can be bilateral
Spread of pain	Variable
Associated symptoms	Nausea, vomiting, photophobia, phonophobia, neck stiffness
Aggravating factors	Physical activity
Relieving factors	Keeping still, vomiting, sleep

Migraine

Recurrent episodic headaches lasting 4–72 hours associated with photophobia, nausea and disability in an otherwise well person are pathognomonic of migraine (Table 9.2). Trigger factors include lack of food, dehydration, oversleeping or lack of sleep and menstruation. Symptomatic treatment of attacks includes non-opioid analgesics, prokinetic antiemetics and triptans, which should be limited to a maximum of 2–3 treatment days a week (10–15 days per month). Prophylaxis should be considered when attacks are frequent and/or fail to respond to symptomatic management.

Tension-type headache

The headache lacks the characteristic associated features of migraine and can occur daily (Table 9.3). Regular exercise and lifestyle change, including biofeedback and cognitive behavioural therapy (CBT), may help associated stress. Symptomatic treatment with non-opioid analgesics is appropriate for episodic attacks occurring on fewer than two days per week. Amitriptyline, 10–150 mg daily, is indicated for chronic tension-type headache.

Cluster headache

This is frequently misdiagnosed as migraine despite stereotypical symptoms (Table 9.4). Prophylaxis is the mainstay of management. First line prophylaxis is verapamil, 240–960 mg in three

Table 9.3 Characteristics of tension-type headache.

Prevalence	2 in 3
Male:female ratio	4:5
Age group most affected	30–40 years
Frequency of attacks	Episodic (<15 days per month); chronic (≥15 days per month)
Duration of attacks	30 minutes to days
Intensity of pain	Mild or moderate
Quality of pain	Pressing, tightening, non-pulsating
Site of pain	Bilateral
Spread of pain	Variable
Associated symptoms	± pericranial tenderness, stress
Aggravating factors	None
Relieving factors	Analgesics (unless medication overuse)

divided daily dosages. Cardiac conduction problems affect about 20% of cluster headache patients taking verapamil and are neither duration- nor dose-dependent. Electrocardiograms (ECGs) to assess PR interval prolongation should be undertaken at baseline, prior to each dose increment, and at six monthly intervals during long-term treatment. Acute treatment includes oxygen (100% at 7 l/min for 10–15 minutes at onset of attack), subcutaneous or intranasal triptans. Analgesics are ineffective and should not be prescribed.

Medication overuse headache

Medication overuse headache (MOH) affects people with a history of a primary headache that has become more frequent. MOH should always be excluded in anyone using symptomatic treatments for headache more often than two to three days a week. It is an avoidable cause of treatment failure, as headache becomes resistant to all lines of management until symptomatic drugs are withdrawn. Drug withdrawal may in itself resolve headache frequency and residual headache can be treated more effectively,

Temporomandibular disorders (TMD)

The natural history of TMD is extremely variable. About 25% of sufferers are likely to be disabled by the pain. Depression and somatisation are the best predictors of chronicity. The diagnosis is clinical, based on history (Table 9.5) and examination. The majority of patients have myofascial pain and disorders of the joint itself are rare. It is essential that TMD patients have a careful assessment, which includes psychosocial factors and takes into account the presence of other chronic pain sites. The small minority of patients that cannot be managed by careful explanation and education may benefit from physiotherapy and cognitive behaviour therapy

Table 9.4 Characteristics of cluster headache.

Prevalence	1 in 1000
Male:female ratio	3.5–7:1
Age group most affected	30–40 years
Frequency of attacks	One on alternate days up to eight per day. These occur over 6–8 weeks usually at the same time each year (episodic) or continuous with remission no longer than a month each year (chronic)
Duration of attacks	15–180 minutes
Intensity of pain	Severe or excruciating
Quality of pain	Sudden, sharp, stabbing, burning, superficial
Site of pain	Unilateral orbital, supraorbital or temporal
Spread of pain	Non-radiating
Associated symptoms	Restlessness and agitation. Ipsilateral symptoms of conjunctival injection and/or lacrimation, nasal congestion and/or rhinorrhoea
Aggravating factors	Alcohol, histamine, glyceryl trinitrate, sleep
Relieving factors	None

Table 9.5 Characteristics of temporomandibular disorders.

Prevalence	1 in 8–10
Male:female ratio	Male ≪ female
Age group most affected	30–50 years
Frequency of attacks	Daily
Duration of attacks	Continuous or intermittent – can be worse on waking or by evening
Intensity of pain	Mild to moderate
Quality of pain	Dull, aching, throbbing
Site of pain	Periauricular and associated muscles
Spread of pain	Temple, neck
Associated symptoms	Decreased mouth opening, bruxism, anxiety, other bodily pains
Aggravating factors	Jaw movement, eating, stress
Relieving factors	Jaw rest

(CBT). Although studies have shown that ibuprofen with diazepam or diazepam alone can be effective for acute episodes, treatment with amitriptyline, 10–150 mg daily, is the recommended medical management for intractable cases. There is insufficient evidence either for or against the use of stabilisation splint therapy over other active interventions for the treatment of TMD but there is some weak evidence that these splints can reduce pain severity. However, occlusal rehabilitation neither treats nor prevents TMD.

Trigeminal neuralgia

Patients with classical trigeminal neuralgia report a sharp shooting, electric shock like pain that lasts for a few seconds and may recur many times a day. After months or weeks a period of complete pain remission may result that can last weeks or months. The second and/or third divisions of the fifth cranial nerve are affected in 85% of cases. It is important to note whether the pain is evoked by light touch activities and/or whether it occurs spontaneously, as drugs may be more effective in reducing the number of spontaneous attacks in these cases. The diagnosis is clinical, based on history (Table 9.6) and examination. Sensory testing will potentially differentiate between symptomatic and idiopathic trigeminal neuralgia but is not available in all centres. Carbamazepine, 400–1200 mg, is the first line drug but should be changed to oxcarbazepine, 300–1200 mg, as soon as it loses efficacy or becomes poorly tolerated. Patients should be referred early for a neurosurgical opinion and in those who are medically fit and have an identifiable compression on MRI, microvascular decompression is the most satisfactory procedure when performed by a skilled neurosurgeon. International guidelines have been published.

Persistent idiopathic facial pain

Previously known as atypical facial pain, this condition is postulated to be of psychogenic origin but there may be vascular or neurological causes. The diagnosis is often a diagnosis of exclusion, based on history (Table 9.7) and examination. There is no

Table 9.6 Characteristics of trigeminal neuralgia.

Prevalence	1 in 20 000
Male:female ratio	2:3
Age group most affected	>50 years
Frequency of attacks	Episodic paroxysms
Duration of attacks	Seconds to less than two minutes
Intensity of pain	Severe
Quality of pain	Sudden, shooting, stabbing, superficial
Site of pain	Unilateral in distribution of trigeminal nerve mainly second and third division
Spread of pain	Other divisions of trigeminal nerve
Associated symptoms	Loss of weight, depression
Aggravating factors	Trigger points, eating, talking, washing the face, cleaning teeth
Relieving factors	Avoiding trigger factors

Table 9.7 Characteristics of persistent idiopathic facial pain.

Prevalence	unknown
Male:female ratio	Male < female
Age group most affected	40-50 years
Frequency of attacks	Daily, but can have prolonged pain-free periods
Duration of attacks	Continuous
Intensity of pain	Mild to severe, but not unbearable
Quality of pain	Throbbing, deep, diffuse, boring, nagging
Site of pain	Deep non-muscular areas of the face, initially unilateral, does not follow nerve distribution
Spread of pain	Poorly localised
Associated symptoms	Life events, anxiety, depression, other bodily pains
Aggravating factors	Stress, fatigue, no trigger points
Relieving factors	Rest

sensory loss or other physical sign. Patients with persistent idiopathic pain need to be assessed carefully, which includes eliciting their treatment goals and beliefs about treatments. One-quarter of sufferers reported co-morbid irritable bowel syndrome, chronic fatigue and chronic widespread pain. In line with other chronic pain conditions, unnecessary investigations and treatments make pain intractable and results in depressed patients. Clinicians often feel less optimistic about their ability to manage these patients successfully. A biopsychosocial approach to treatment is needed and, in those who are found to have a high index of disability, CBT should be combined with drugs. The SSRI'S (fluoxetine 20 mg daily) are associated with fewer side effects than tricyclics (nortyptyline, 10–40 mg, or dosulepin, 75 mg, daily) but may be less effective in pain relief.

Further reading

Gronseth, G, Cruccu, G, Alksne, J, Argoff, C, Brainin, M, Burchiel, K *et al.* (2008) Practice parameter: the diagnostic evaluation and treatment of trigeminal neuralgia (an evidence-based review): report of the Quality Standards Subcommittee of the American Academy of Neurology and the European Federation of Neurological Societies. *Neurology*, **71** (15), 1183–1190.

Headache Classification Subcommittee of the International Headache Society (IHS) (2004) The International Classification of Headache Disorders (2nd edition). *Cephalalgia*, **24** (suppl 1):1–160. Available from: www.i-h-s.org.

MacGregor, A & Frith, A (eds) (2008) *ABC of Headache*. Oxford: Blackwell Publishing Ltd.

MacGregor, EA, Steiner, TJ & Davies, PTG (2010) *Guidelines for All Healthcare Professionals in the Diagnosis and Management of Migraine, Tension-Type, Cluster and Medication-Overuse Headache*. Available at: http://www.bash.org.uk.

Olesen, J, Goadsby, PJ, Ramadan, N, Tfelt-Hansen, P & Welch, KMA (eds) (2005) *The Headaches*, 3rd edn. Philadelphia, PA: Lippincott Williams and Wilkins.

Zakrzewska, JM (Ed.) (2008) *Orofacial Pain*. Oxford: Oxford University Press.

Further resources

Professional organisation

British Association for the Study of Headache, c/o Dr Fayyaz Ahmed, Department of Neurology, Hull Royal Infirmary, Analby Road, Hull HU3 2JZ, UK. Web site: www.bash.org.uk.

Lay organisations

Brain and Spine Helpline, 3.36 Canterbury Court, Kennington Park, 1–3 Brixton Road, London SW9 6DE, UK. Helpline: 0808 808 1000. Web site: www.brainandspine.org.uk.

Migraine Action Association, 27 East Street, Leicester, LE1 6NB, UK. Web site: www.migraine.org.uk.

Ouch (UK): The Organisation for the Understanding of Cluster Headache, PO Box 62, Tenby SA70 9AG, UK. Helpline: 01646 651 979. Web site: www.ouchuk.org.

The Migraine Trust, 52–53 Russell Square, London WC1B 4HP, UK. Web site: www.migrainetrust.org.

Trigeminal Neuralgia Association (TNA UK), PO Box 234, Oxted RH8 8BE, UK. Web site: www.tna.org.uk.

CHAPTER 10

Cancer Pain

Marie Fallon

Edinburgh Cancer Research Centre, University of Edinburgh, UK

OVERVIEW

- The management of cancer pain is clearly an important, although not exclusive, part of palliative care
- The integration of cancer pain management into broader therapeutic strategies which encompass palliative care is widely accepted as optimum practice
- Cancer encompasses a range of illnesses on a background of varying co-morbidities and a multitude of tumoricidal strategies; such strategies have been increasing exponentially over the last decade and this, in turn, leads to the development of new side effects which also need to be managed
- Several cancers are now regarded as 'chronic illnesses' because of improved palliative tumoricidal treatments

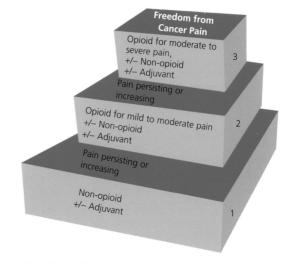

Figure 10.1 WHO ladder for cancer pain relief. (Source: http://www.who.int/cancer/palliative/painladder/en/. Accessed 28/10/11. Reproduced with permission from WHO.)

Introduction

Cancer pain assessment clearly has to encompass both an accurate assessment of the pain and take into account the underlying disease, as well as past, current and proposed treatment. The WHO analgesic ladder (Figure 10.1) when applied appropriately can achieve good pain control in the majority of patients. There are, however, major differences in how it is used and in the resultant outcomes. The principles of the analgesic ladder are as follows:

1. choose step depending on severity of pain;
2. add an adjuvant depending on underlying pain mechanisms;
3. use a non-steroidal depending on risk versus benefit;
4. prescribe regular medication *and* allow 'as required' medication for breakthrough pain.

Generally the evidence for opioids and adjuvant analgesics points to co-prescribing, usually resulting in a reduction in the opioid dose required (Table 10.1).

The mainstay for pharmacological management of cancer pain is opioid based. The pure mu agonists are recommended. The constant continuing challenge with opioids for all clinicians managing patients with cancer pain is to find the optimum balance between

Table 10.1 Areas where adjuvant analgesics may be useful.

Type of pain	Agents with evidence for use
Neuropathic Pain	Antidepressants: *Despiramine, amitriptyline, duloxetine*
	Anticonvulsants: *Gabapentin, Pregabalin*
Bone pain	*Bisphosphonates, radiopharmaceuticals*
Bowel obstruction	*Anticholinergic drugs, somatostatin analogue*
Multiple use	*Dexamethasone*

the desired effect of pain relief and the undesired common side effects. This aim will encompass finding the appropriate opioid and route for the individual patient and appropriate provision for so-called 'breakthrough' medication. Anticipatory management of all the common opioid side effects is critical, along with regular assessment to detect early signs of emerging side effects, heralding opioid toxicity (Figure 10.2). Opioid-induced toxicity can have a significant impact on quality of life and arguably, if undetected, quantity of life. Opioid-induced hyperalgesia has been evaluated in both the laboratory and in early situations in the clinic. Following early debate as to the existence of this phenomenon, it is generally

ABC of Pain, First edition. Edited by Lesley A Colvin and Marie Fallon.

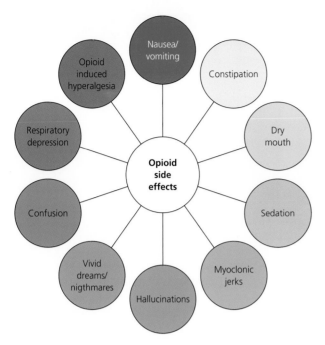

Figure 10.2 Opioid-related side effects.

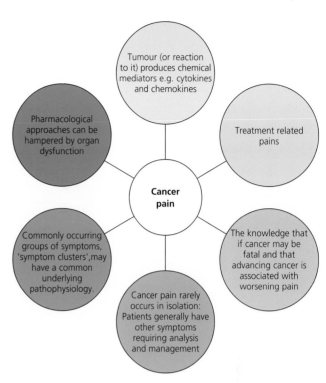

Figure 10.3 Many complex additional factors need to be considered in cancer pain management.

agreed that this does exist as a specific phenomenon and can be part of the spectrum of opioid toxicity described already or occur by itself. It certainly should be considered in any patient, particularly on a background of rapid escalation of opioid dose where there is widespread sensitivity in the skin.

The optimum balance with opioids in cancer pain management is achieved with the use of other appropriate drugs and the category of drugs known as the adjuvant analgesics plays a key role in cancer pain management.

Cancer pain versus non-malignant pain

Pain due to cancer can be considered as the spectrum of pains covered in this book but with the addition of five key important factors, as outlined in Figure 10.3. Treatment-related pain can be particularly challenging. Patients may not complain of even very severe pains related to treatment, because of the context in which they are experiencing the pain. Treatment-related challenging pains include chemotherapy-induced peripheral neuropathy, hormone and chemotherapy-related arthropathy, radio- and chemotherapy-related mucositosis, radiation burns and idiosynchratic peripheral nerve pains with newer treatments, including monoclonal antibodies

Assessment

The principles of pain assessment clearly apply to cancer pain; however, knowledge of the following is important:

1 Common cancer pain syndromes, for example Pancoast's tumour with brachial plexopathy (Figure 10.4), pelvic disease and lumbo-sacral plexopathy, patterns of visceral pain due to liver (Figure 10.5), pancreatic, bladder disease.

2 Some pains can herald acute problems needing urgent management, such as escalating radicular back pain with spinal cord compression (Figure 10.6) and headache and vomiting with raised intracranial pressure.

3 Pain can often herald recurrent or further advancing cancer before it is obvious on imaging, including MRI, CT or even occasionally PET scanning. On the other hand, bone metastases can be present on radioisotope scan or even plain X-ray (Figure 10.7) and be asymptomatic.

With the background knowledge of common patterns of disease spread and cancer pain syndromes, the key to cancer pain assessment is active, attentive listening and appropriate physical examination and imaging as/if appropriate. The multifactorial influences such as sleep deprivation, anxiety, fear and depression will, of course, amplify input to the spinal cord and should be considered as such, rather than simply worsening patients' coping ability with pain only existing in a parallel system (Figure 10.8). Clearly removal of pain from the clinical picture will not always result in resolution of 'distress'.

Management of cancer pain

Management of cancer pain is based on an interdisciplinary approach that should involve an appropriate combination of professionals which will vary between patients. It is, however, important that it is clear who is coordinating care, and that communication is effective. It is usual for the focus of care to shift and the person coordinating that care also to shift at different points in a cancer illness.

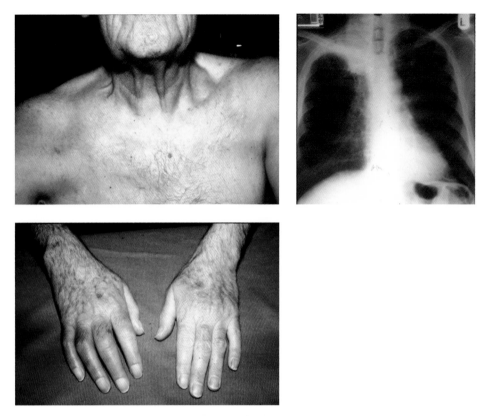

Figure 10.4 Pancoast's tumour may present with supraclavicular swelling and a brachial plexopathy.

Opioid responsiveness

Opioid responsiveness is a continuum and is usually a retrospective diagnosis. It is true that some pain syndromes are less likely to be opioid responsive and this is particularly true of cancer-related neuropathic pain and bone pain. It is also true that many difficult to manage cancer pains are of mixed aetiology. In neuropathic pain the dose of opioid required to control pain is often associated with unacceptable side effects. Cancer-induced bone pain (CIBP) has three main clinical components: background pain, spontaneous pain at rest and pain induced by a particular event, for example walking, coughing. Only the background component of CIBP responds easily to opioids while the spontaneous and activity-related components present a management challenge. Both spontaneous pain and activity-related pain can have peaked and resolved before any standard oral opioid preparation could possibly have an analgesic effect. The faster acting oral and nasal fentanyl preparations may be useful here. If, however, the breakthrough pain has resolved by 10 minutes, even the newer fentanyl preparations are unlikely to be useful. The role of adjuvant analgesics in CIBP is under clinical investigation after promising preclinical work with gabapentin.

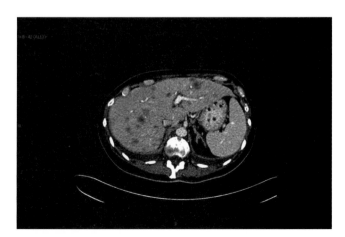

Figure 10.5 Computed tomogram of enlarged liver due to metastatic spread of cancer.

Strategies to improve opioid responsiveness

Therapeutic options

Opening the 'therapeutic window'

- More aggressive side-effect treatment, for example a psychostimulant for sedation.
- Aggressive management of other co-existing symptoms, such as constipation and nausea.

Identifying an opioid with a more favourable balance between analgesia and side effects (Opioid switch)

It is clear that because of unpredictable genetic variations in both opioid analgesia and susceptibility to opioid side effects, patients who fail to respond to the first opioid prescribed should be given a trial of another opioid(s). In cancer pain management, methadone is often prescribed for patients who fail on other opioids. Methadone has unusual properties, including increased potency on chronic dosing and as the dose increases, therefore, a sliding scale conversion is used. In addition, it has a variable half-life, meaning that steady state can be reached in a few days or a few weeks! The equianalgesic conversion table gives a suggested dose conversion, but should always remain for guidance only (Box 10.3).

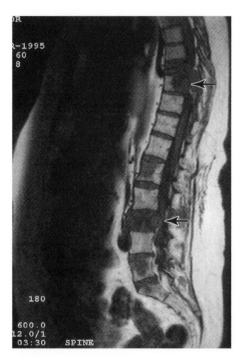

Figure 10.6 Magnetic resonance image showing patient with spinal cord compression at two different sites (arrows).

Pharmacological techniques to reduce systemic opioid requirement

There is a range of techniques that should be considered in order to minimise opioid dose and maximise pain relief (Figure 10.9). Some of these will require close communication with other members of the team, such as the oncologist and pain specialist anaesthetist. Particularly where neuraxial infusions are being considered, it is important to define the aims of treatment and ensure that if analgesia is improved there are systems in place to allow the patient to gain maximum benefit from this.

Non-pharmacological techniques to reduce systemic opioid requirements

While multimodal pharmacological strategies can reduce opioid requirements markedly, there is a range of other approaches that

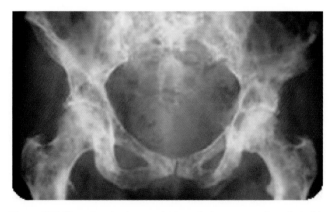

Figure 10.7 X-ray showing bone metastases that were asymptomatic in this patient.

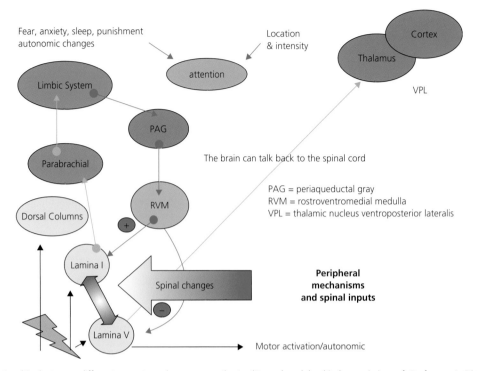

Figure 10.8 Interrelationship between different symptoms in cancer patients. (Reproduced by kind permission of Professor A Dickenson, Professor of Neuropharmacology, University College, London, UK.)

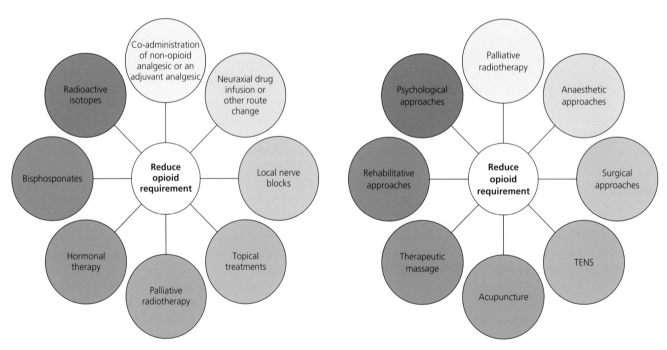

Figure 10.9 Pharmacological strategies to reduce systemic opioid requirements.

Figure 10.10 Non-pharmacological strategies to reduce opioid requirements.

need to be considered as part of an overall multidisciplinary management plan (Figure 10.10). Simple techniques such as a TENS machine can be effective in providing additional pain relief and may give the patient some degree of control. Surgical approaches such as spinal stabilisation, are evolving and the use of vertebroplasty has become more common.

Special considerations

1 Several palliative chemotherapy scenarios are likely to control visceral disease but not bone disease. This, therefore, can mean prolongation of life with worsening uncontrolled bone pain.

2 In breast and prostate cancer where hormone sensitivity exists, a switch in hormone can result in renewed control of bone pain within weeks.

3 Some metastatic cancers are now chronic illnesses with acute on chronic pain. Prognosis is clearly important in some pain management decisions; however, prognosticating can be challenging. It is known that primary tumour site, performance status and the following parameters are important:

- ↑ C-reactive protein (CRP)
- ↑ Lactate dehydrogenase (LDG)
- ↑ white cell count
- ↑ albumin

CRP is a clinical biomarker for interleukin-6 (I-L6). I-L6 is a strong indicator of systemic inflammation, heralds a poor prognosis and is commonly associated with pain and linked to the pain, fatigue, depression cluster.

Newer treatments

There are a number of novel therapies emerging that may be useful additions to the pharmacological armamentarium for management of cancer pain. These include:

- Oxycodone:naloxone (Targinact®). This preparation relies on the formulation of the medication such that the naloxone is retained within the gastrointestinal tract and, having a higher mu opioid receptor affinity, binds to the mu opioid receptor. This blocks the oxycodone from binding to the opioid receptors within the gut and should thus reduce opioid related GI side effects, such as constipation, while maintaining the systemic analgesic effects of oxycodone. It is available in both short and long acting preparations.
- Opioid combinations such as morphine/oxycodone (Moxduo®) are in the early stages of development, but preliminary evidence indicates that by using a synergistic action between different opioids, the side effect profile can be reduced.
- Tapentadol acts at the mu opioid receptor and also at the noradrenaline receptor, and may thus have a potential role in cancer pain, where there is often a neuropathic component.

- 8% Capsaicin patch – this is described in more detail in Chapter 5. It is licensed for neuropathic pain and has been used for chemotherapy-induced peripheral neuropathy but it is unknown as yet if will be of benefit in cancer-related peripheral neuropathic pain
- Cannabinoids – Sativex® oromucosal spray – this is available for relief of spasticity in multiple sclerosis and there are continuing trials to define its use in cancer pain following promising results in phase II studies.

Summary

Cancer pain is common at all stages of the disease, and is feared by sufferers and carers. Additionally, pain related to cancer treatment is an increasing problem as survival improves and oncological therapies expand. The key to successful management is careful assessment (and reassessment) with close communication between different team members. A wider range of pharmacological treatments is available, with opioids remaining the mainstay of treatment. New strategies may help to improve problems with side effects. Using multimodal pharmacological techniques in combination with a range of non-pharmacological options gives the best chance of managing pain successfully. Other symptoms co-exist commonly and should be managed in parallel.

Further reading

European Journal of Cancer (2008) Special Issue: Palliative Medicine – the Art ad the Science. *European Journal of Cancer*, **44** (8).

Fallon, MT & Hanks, GW (eds) (2006) *ABC of Palliative Care*, 2nd edn. BMJ/Blackwell Publishing Ltd.

Hanks, G, Cherny, N, Kaasa, S, Portenoy, R, Christakis, N & Fallon, M (eds) (2009) *Oxford Textbook of Palliative Medicine*, 4th edn. Oxford: Oxford University Press.

Palliative Medicine (2011) Special Issue: The Supporting Evidence (Systematic Reviews) for the updated 2011 EAPC guidelines on opioids for cancer pain. *Palliative Medicine*, **25** (5).

CHAPTER 11

Treating Pain in Patients with Drug-dependence Problems

Jane C Ballantyne

Department of Anesthesiology and Pain Medicine, University of Washington, Seattle, WA, USA

OVERVIEW

- Pre-existing substance dependence does not preclude use of opioids for pain, but does complicate opioid use
- Substance dependence virtually never arises *de novo* during the treatment of acute pain, or pain at the end of life
- Substance dependence can interfered seriously with opioid treatment of chronic pain
- Both existing substance dependence and assessed risk of substance dependence warrant careful and structured chronic opioid pain management
- Structured chronic opioid pain management can include use of written consents or agreements, urine testing, regular visits and prescription pick-ups, and good communication between pharmacists and prescribers

---

Introduction

Reasonably one can be concerned in patients with known drug dependence that their dependence will interfere with pain treatment, particularly treatment of pain with opioids. Concerns centre mainly on fears of addiction relapse when patients are given addictive drugs in the medical setting, but there may also be issues with drug interactions, with dosing for active users or with drug seeking for recreational use. Drug dependence does not preclude using addictive drugs during medical treatment of pain, but it does introduce several complications that must be considered when treating these patients. The acute pain, pain at the end of life and chronic pain situations are different, and are treated as separate entities in this chapter. The chapter focuses on dependence during chronic pain treatment, since this is where most of the complexities of concurrent pain and substance dependence arise.

Defining addiction

Much effort has been placed towards developing uniform criteria and descriptors for addiction, so that it becomes a recognised medical condition and patients with addiction can thereby gain

access to addiction treatment. These efforts have culminated in the American Psychiatric Association's DSM IV criteria (Table 11.1), reflected also in the ICD-10 and WHO classifications of addiction and addiction terminology, which use the term 'substance dependence' to denote what would in general parlance be termed 'drug addiction'. Unfortunately, although the definitions did satisfy the need to medicalise addiction, it later became difficult to define and identify addiction in patients treated with opioids for pain, because these patients develop opioid dependence without necessarily reaching the criteria for addiction. This has produced much confusion and a great deal of difficulty in defining addiction and assessing addiction rates in opioid treated pain patients, to the extent that as new criteria are being developed in DSM V the word, dependence, will be dropped.

For the purposes of this chapter, it should be considered that 'substance dependence' describes patients who reach DSM IV criteria for substance dependence (addiction), which includes drug tolerance, drug dependence (manifest as withdrawal when drug is tapered or withdrawn) and at least one of the aberrant behaviours described by criteria. It is important to note here that all patients treated chronically with opioids may demonstrate opioid tolerance and dependence, but unless they also exhibit opioid seeking behaviours, such as compulsive use and craving, they do not meet the criteria for addiction (Table 11.2).

Treating acute pain

It is safe to say that addiction virtually never develops *de novo* from opioid treatment of acute pain. The exception might be the case when acute pain progresses through subacute pain to chronic pain, and opioid use becomes long term rather than short term. Provided opioid use is structured and supervised, as it usually is in the acute pain setting, particularly when treating post-operative or post-trauma pain, addiction rarely develops. There may be a concern, however, in patients who already carry a current or past substance dependence diagnosis, that opioid treatment of pain could trigger a worsening or relapse of the condition. When a patient with a substance dependence diagnosis expresses such concern it may be helpful to avoid opioids or other addictive medications (e.g. benzodiazepines) wherever possible.

In general, the principle of management of acute pain in substance-dependent patients is to treat pain using whatever

---

ABC of Pain, First edition. Edited by Lesley A Colvin and Marie Fallon.

Table 11.1 DSM IV Substance abuse and dependence criteria.

DSM-IV Substance Abuse Criteria	
A. A maladaptive pattern of substance use leading to clinically significant impairment or distress, as manifested by one (or more) of the following, occurring within a 12-month period:	• recurrent substance use resulting in a failure to fulfill major role obligations at work, school or home • recurrent substance use in situations in which it is physically hazardous • recurrent substance-related legal problems • continued substance use despite having persistent or recurrent social or interpersonal problems caused or exacerbated by the effects of the substance
B. The symptoms have never met the criteria for Substance Dependence for this class of substance	

DSM-IV Substance Dependence Criteria	
Addiction (termed *substance dependence* by the American Psychiatric Association) is a maladaptive pattern of substance use leading to clinically significant impairment or distress, as manifested by one (or more) of the following, occurring within a 12-month period:	• *Tolerance*, as defined by either of the following: (a) A need for markedly increased amount of the substance to achieve intoxication or the desired effect or (b) Markedly diminished effect with continued use of the same amount of the substance • *Withdrawal*, as manifested by either of the following: (a) The characteristic withdrawal syndrome for the substance or (b) the same (or closely related) substance is taken to relieve or avoid withdrawal symptoms • The substance is often taken in larger amounts or over a longer period than intended. • There is a persistent desire or unsuccessful efforts to cut down or control substance use. • A great deal of time is spent in activities necessary to obtain the substance, use the substance, or recover from its effects. • Important social, occupational, or recreational activities are given up or reduced because of substance use. • The substance use is continued despite knowledge of having a persistent physical or psychological problem that is likely to have been caused or exacerbated by the substance (for example, current cocaine use despite recognition of cocaine-induced depression or continued drinking despite recognition that an ulcer was made worse by alcohol consumption)
Substance dependence may be:	• with physiologic dependence (evidence of tolerance or withdrawal) or • without physiologic dependence (no evidence of tolerance or withdrawal)

Source: American Psychiatric Association (1994) *Diagnostic and Statistical Manual of Mental Disorders*, 4th edn. Washington, DC: American Psychiatric Association.

NOTE: Unlike the criteria for Substance Dependence, the criteria for Substance Abuse do not include tolerance, withdrawal or a pattern of compulsive use, and instead include only the harmful consequences of repeated use. The term *abuse* should be applied only to a pattern of substance use that meets the criteria for this disorder; the term should not be used as a synonym for 'use', 'misuse', or 'hazardous use'. The term will not often apply to opioid-treated pain patients who generally receive continuous opioid treatment, and therefore develop tolerance and dependence.

treatment best relieves the pain, including using opioids as needed. The acute pain setting is not the right setting for initiating or continuing active addiction treatment, but when known substance abusers are under care, plans should be made for addiction treatment after the acute pain episode. A number of drug interactions may arise during surgery and anaesthesia, and during acute pain treatment, when substance dependence is active; these are summarised in Table 11.3. In particular, substance-dependent patients using opioids will manifest tolerance as resistance to opioids, and the need to use large opioid doses to achieve analgesia. Another feature of chronic opioid use is a narrowing of the therapeutic window, reducing the safety margin and risking respiratory depression despite inadequate analgesia. This makes it advisable to maximise the use of non-opioid pain interventions, such as neuraxial and regional anesthesia and non-steroidal anti-inflammatory drugs (NSAIDs), to obviate the need for opioids wherever possible.

Palliative care

The palliative care setting, or the care of patients at the end of life, is another setting where concerns about addiction are few. The absolute goal of palliative care at the end of life is comfort, so that even if addictive behaviours persist during terminal illness, they are generally tolerated (Figure 11.1). In fact, it is extremely rare for addictive behaviours to persist because adjustments to terminal illness generally predominate. As with acute pain, pain at the end of life can be treated with whatever means are needed to provide pain and symptom relief for the dying patient, and it would never be appropriate to withhold opioids because of a past or present history of substance dependence. Again, there may be resistance to opioids necessitating high doses to achieve adequate analgesia, and the use of non-opioid analgesics and other interventions should be maximised to achieve the best comfort possible.

Treating chronic pain

Universal precautions and triage

Chronic pain is common, yet not all patients with chronic pain seek medical treatment of their pain. The factors that lead patients to seek help for their chronic pain are many but, in some cases, may place the patients at particular risk of developing substance dependence, and arguably should therefore be treated with special caution (Box 11.1).

Table 11.2 Definitions related to the use of opioids for the treatment of pain.

I Addiction

Addiction is a primary, chronic, neurobiologic disease, with genetic, psychosocial, and environmental factors influencing its development and manifestations. It is characterized by behaviours that include one or more of the following: impaired control over drug use, compulsive use, continued use despite harm, and craving.

II Physical Dependence

Physical dependence is a state of adaptation that is manifested by a drug class specific withdrawal syndrome that can be produced by abrupt cessation, rapid dose reduction, decreasing blood level of the drug, and/or administration of an antagonist.

III Tolerance

Tolerance is a state of adaptation in which exposure to a drug induces changes that result in a diminution of one or more of the drug's effects over time.

Source: Savage, S, Covington, EC, Ehit, HA, Hunt, J, Joranson, D& Schnoll, SH (2001)*Definitions related to the use of opioids for the treatment of pain*. A Consensus Document From the American Academy of Pain Medicine, the American Pain Society, and the American Society of Addiction Medicine.

Box 11.1 **Chronic pain + risk of substance dependence – Common patient profile**

- Personality disorder
- Anxiety/depression
- Somatization
- History of childhood abuse

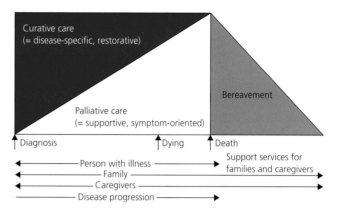

Figure 11.1 A model for palliative and curative care.

Gourlay and Heit described the concept of 'universal precautions' applied to all patients treated with opioids for chronic pain, whereby all patients should be considered at risk of developing addiction, and should therefore be screened carefully and monitored before and during treatment (Table 11.4). Screening can help triage patients to a level of care that is suitable according to their level of risk. For example, high risk patients ideally should be treated in a multidisciplinary setting whereas low risk patients could be safely treated in the primary care setting with minimal precautions. Known past or present substance dependence automatically places patients in the high risk category for worsening or relapse of substance dependence.

Screening

There are a number of validated addiction screening instruments developed for the chronic pain treatment setting, some elaborate

Table 11.3 Drug interactions and other problems during active substance use.

Drug	Problems and interactions
Alcohol	*Acute intoxication* Effects of opioids and hypnotics enhanced. Caution with dosage. Will have delayed gastric emptying. *Chronic use* Full work up needed to identify alcohol related disease. Hepatic enzyme induction results in tolerance to effects of opioids and hypnotics. May need increased anesthetic doses.
Marijuana	Easy to detect because of slow elimination (up to one week). Tachycardia associated with chronic or moderate use. Hypotension and bradycardia associated with toxicity. Chronic smoking produces lung disease.
Cocaine	Interferes with presynaptic uptake of sympathomimetic neurotransmitters producing excitatory state. Rapid metabolism, but inactive metabolites can be detected late. Toxicity (overdose) can result in cardiac death.
Heroin	Opioid tolerance.
Hallucinogens and 'club drugs'	During use, high risk of autonomic dysregulation and coronary or cerebral vascular spasm. Overdose can kill through respiratory depression, siezures and coma. May be exaggerated obtundation with opioids. Cardiomyopathy may develop in repeat users.
Lysergic acid diethylamide (LSD) 3,4-methylenedioxmethamphetamine (MDMA),'ecstasy'	Water hunger can lead to cerebral/pulmonary edema.
Gamma-hydroxybutyrate (GHB),'liquid ecstasy'	Difficult to detect because rapidly eliminated.
Solvents	Toxicity produces possible cardiac dysrythmias, pulmonary/hepatic toxicity, cerebral/pulmonary edema. Chronic use can cause CNS degeneration or diffuse brain atrophy.

Source: Ballantyne, JC (2008) Psychiatric disease, chronic pain and substance abuse. In:Sweitzer, B-J (ed.)*Handbook of Preoperative Assessment and Managment*, 2nd edn. Philadelphia, PA:Lippincott Williams and Wilkins.

Table 11.4 The ten principles of 'universal precautions'.

1 Diagnosis with appropriate differential
2 Psychological assessment including risk of addictive disorders
3 Informed consent (verbal or written/signed)
4 Treatment agreement (verbal or written/signed)
5 Pre/post intervention assessment of pain level and function
6 Appropriate trial of opioid therapy +/–adjunctive medication
7 Reassessment of pain score and level of function
8 Regularly assess the 'Four A's'of pain medicine: *Analgesia, Activity, Adverse reactions and Aberrant behaviour*
9 Periodically review pain and comorbidity diagnoses, including addictive disorders
10 Documentation

Adapted from Gourlay, D, Heit, H &Almarhezi,A (2005)Universal Precautions in Pain Medicine: A rational approach to the management of chronic pain.*Pain Medicine*, **6**(2), 107–112.

Table 11.5 Commonly used opioid risk screening instruments.

	Butler et al.	Screener and Opioid Assessment for Patients with Pain (SOAPP). 5, 14 or 24-item questionnaire. Completed by patients.
2005	Webster & Webster	Opioid Risk Tool (ORT). 5-item questionnaire. Completed by patients.
2005	Passik et al.	Pain Assessment and Documentation Tool (PADT). Assesses fourdomains. Completed by physicians.
2006	Belgrade et al.	Scoring system to predict outcome (DIRE) Assesses fourdomains (diagnosis, intractability, risk, efficacy). Completed by physicians.
2007	Butler et al.	Current Opioid Misuse Measure (COMM) 17-item questionnaire. Complete by patients.

Butler, SF, Budman, SH, Fernandez, K&., Jamison, RN (2004) Validation of a screener and opioid assessment measure for patients with chronic pain. *Pain, 112*, 65–75.
Webster, L& Webster, R (2005) Predicting aberrant behaviors in opioid-treated patients: preliminary validation of the Opioid Risk Tool. *Pain Med.*, **6**(6), 432–442.
Passik, SD, Kirsh, KL, Whitcomb, L, et al. (2005) Monitoring outcomes during long-term opioid therapy for noncancer pain: results with the Pain Assessment and Documentation Tool. *J Opioid Manag*, **1**(5), 257–266.
Belgrade, MJ, Schamber, CD, Lindgren, BR (2006) The DIRE score: Predicting outcomes of opioid prescribing for chronic pain. *J Pain*, **7**(9), 671–681.
Butler, SF, Budman, SH, Fernandez, KC, et al.(2007) Development and validation of the Current Opioid Misuse Measure. *Pain*, **130**(1–2): 144–156.

and others simple. Table 11.5 lists some of the more commonly used screening instruments. Since use of screening instruments places a burden on busy practices, these instruments have tended to become ever more simple and brief to make them practical and usable. The Opioid Risk Tool (ORT) has just eight simple questions filled out by the physician or patient and calculates a score to indicate level of risk (Table 11.6). The Screener and Opioid Assessment for Patients with Pain (SOAPP) is more elaborate but is now available in a brief form that increases its utility in clinical practice. Once risk is calculated using a screening instrument, it can then be balanced against calculated benefit in a risk: benefit assessment, and for *high risk:low benefit* patients it may be better to advise against using opioids for pain.

Table 11.6 Stratifying Risk: Opioid Risk Tool.

		Female	Male
• Five-question clinical interview to assess patients			
• Specifically developed to screen patients with chronic pain who will be using opioids	**Family history of substance abuse**		
• Quantifies the level of risk for patient	Alcohol	[ ] 1	[ ] 3
• Three risk categories	Illegal drugs	[ ] 2	[ ] 3
○ Low: 0–3 points	Prescription drugs	[ ] 4	[ ] 4
○ Moderate: 4–7 points			
○ High: 8 points and above	**Personal history of substance abuse**		
	Alcohol	[ ] 3	[ ] 3
	Illegal drugs	[ ] 4	[ ] 4
	Prescription drugs	[ ] 5	[ ] 5
	Age (if between 16–45)	[ ] 1	[ ] 1
	History of preadolescent sexual abuse	[ ] 3	[ ] 0
	Psychological disease		
	Attention deficit disorder, obsessive-compulsive disorder, bipolar, schizophrenia	[ ] 2	[ ] 2
	Depression	[ ] 1	[ ] 12
	Scoring Total: _____		

Adapted from Webster, L & Webster, R (2005) Predicting aberrant behaviors in opioid-treated patients: preliminary validation of the Opioid Risk Tool. Pain Med., 6(6), 432–442. align="left"

Consistent use of addiction screening instruments for all patients prescribed opioids for chronic pain may help identify patients who do not otherwise reveal their substance use problem and, provided the instruments are repeated on a regular basis, can also help identify new onset of substance dependence in patients who develop iatrogenic opioid addiction (that is, addiction arising as a direct consequence of opioid treatment of chronic pain).

Opioid agreements

Chronic pain and opioid treatment guidelines may recommend, in addition to screening, use of opioid consents, contracts or agreements. This recommendation is particularly strong for known substance abusers because of their risk of treatment related addiction. The terms 'consent' or 'agreement' are preferred, since the term contract seems legalistic and potentially punitive. Ideally the consent or agreement should inform patients about the benefits and risks of opioid therapy, and provide a means of achieving informed consent. Each practice setting will likely develop its own agreement form according to local preferences, needs and customs. Alternatively, several are available in publications or on the web (Box 11.2) and can be adapted for use in new practice settings.

Box 11.2 **Examples of some websites (URLs) with sample opioid agreements**

www.lni.wa.gov/ClaimsIns/Files/OMD/**agreement**.pdf
www.hendricksonandhunt.com/forms/**opioid agreement**.pdf
www.cpsa.ab.ca/Libraries/Pro TPP/TPP **Sample** Patient_Contract.pdf

(Accessed 7 December 2011)

The agreement used in the author's practice was written in patient friendly language so as to be easily understood by most patients (Figure 11.2).

An important part of the agreement may be to agree on treatment goals, since documentation of treatment goals can be a helpful basis for assessing treatment utility when there seems to be no progress towards reasonable goals, or when aberrant behaviours develop, making it desirable to discontinue the treatment.

Urine testing/toxicology

Several lines of evidence suggest that urine testing should be performed for opioid-treated chronic pain patients. For example, urine testing may pick up 40% more aberrant drug use than could psychometric testing alone. Urine testing can be complicated in terms of choosing the right test and, even more importantly, interpreting the results. Any aberrant value should be verified and confirmed by the testing laboratory, since either absence or presence of a drug may be misleading. For example, oxycodone may be undetectable at low levels, while fentanyl may only be detectable in blood, not urine. Since urine testing is complicated, no attempt is made here to cover the details of urine testing, rather the principles will be outlined.

There is limited evidence as yet supporting urine testing for opioid treated pain patients, and virtually no evidence to guide the

Patient name: _____ Patient DOB: _____ Patient MRN: _____

Opiate Pain Medicine Agreement
(examples of opiates are: hydrocodone, codeine, oxycodone, hydromorphone, morphine, fentanyl)

- ■ If I want to get refills of my pain medicine, I have to come to all of my appointments (at least every 6 months).
- ■ If I miss more than 2 appointments without calling ahead to cancel, my doctor may stop prescribing this medicine for me.
- ■ I cannot get pain medicine from any other doctor or clinic, unless I am in the hospital or my doctor says it is okay.
- ■ I should keep my appointments with other doctors, therapists, and other treatments for my pain in order to get refills of my medicine.
- ■ I will tell my doctor if the medicine is not helping my pain, and will not take more medicine on my own or run out early.
- ■ To get more medicine, I need a paper prescription. These medicines cannot be called into the pharmacy, or filled on a night, holiday, or weekend.
- ■ I may get the prescription from my doctor at my regular appointment, or by calling the practice at least 3 business days before I run out. I may not just walk into the office and ask for a refill.
- ■ I will keep my medicines in a safe place. If my medicine is lost, damaged or stolen, I may not get a new prescription.
- ■ I agree to have a urine drug test at any time. If I don't take the test, I will stop getting the medicine.
- ■ If I share, sell or trade my medicine or use illegal drugs or other pain medicines, my doctor may stop giving me this medicine.
- ■ If I act out at the staff or my doctor, I will not get my medicine, and may be asked to leave the clinic.
- ■ I understand that this medicine may not work for my pain. If this happens, my doctor may stop giving this type of pain medicine to me.
- ■ If I do not follow this agreement, my doctor will stop giving me this type of pain medicine.
- ■ I will get my pain medicine at only one pharmacy.

| Pharmacy _____ | City _____ | Phone _____ |

I have read this agreement, understand it, and will follow it.

Patient Signature _____ Date_____

Physician Signature_____ Date_____

Developed by Robin Canada, David Goldman, Craig Wynn. Department of Medicine, University of Pennsylvania School of Medicine

Figure 11.2 Example Opiate Pain Medicine Agreement.

choice of testing frequency. Patients with known substance abuse would seem the patients most likely to need urine tests as a means of detecting aberrant use since addicts can be deceitful, making urine testing a particularly useful means of detecting misuse and providing support for safe prescribing.

Maintenance versus pain treatment

One final note would be a comment on the situation that substance dependence, or addictive behaviour, is seen to be active during opioid treatment of chronic pain. In this situation, the question that arises is whether opioid treatment should be discontinued or, alternatively, somehow moderated. If, as is often the case, pain relief is questionable, the best course may be to persuade the patient to discontinue opioid pain treatment. This can be a useful approach when the addiction is relatively new in onset and not entrenched or un-eradicable. In most cases, however, an addiction relapse is indicative of a serious and irreversible addiction problem, which may be best treated with opioid maintenance, at least in the case of prescription opioid or heroin addiction. Adequate pain relief could be obtained using maintenance opioids, and the best choice for maintenance treatment of addiction is methadone or buprenorphine. Both are useful analgesics, although for pain treatment they may be used by a different dosing schedule, for example methadone is given 8-hourly rather than the once per day dosing used for addiction maintenance treatment. Buprenorphine has a ceiling effect and is therefore not as effective for severe pain as methadone, which has no ceiling dose.

Whether opioid pain treatment is withdrawn or restructured when addiction emerges, it is vital to include counselling in the plan for continued treatment and treatment of addiction. This should be emphasised particularly, since evidence from opioid maintenance clinics suggests strongly that drug treatment alone is not effective, and that counselling is essential to the success of any addiction treatment.

Conclusion

Known substance dependence complicates pain treatment in several ways, particularly when opioids are needed. In the case of acute pain and pain at the end of life, complications are produced not so much by addiction behaviours per se, but more by a number of drug considerations, including possible drug interactions and, importantly, by opioid tolerance and ineffectiveness for chronic opioid users and abusers. For patients with chronic pain, other important constraints are the risk of addiction re-emerging or worsening, the risk of new onset of opioid addiction (iatrogenic addiction) and the risk of drug getting into the wrong hands (careless or deliberate diversion) when patients are unreliable.

Further reading

American Psychiatric Association (1994) *Diagnostic and Statistical Manual of Mental Disorders*, 4th edn. Washington, DC: American Psychiatric Association.

Ballantyne, JC & LaForge, SL (2007) Opioid dependence and addiction in opioid treated pain patients. *Pain,* **129**, 235–255.

Chou, R, Fanciullo, GJ, Fine, PG, et al. (2009) Clinical guidelines for the use of chronic opioid therapy in chronic noncancer pain. *J Pain,* **10** (2), 113–130.

Heit, HA (2003) Addiction, physical dependence, and tolerance: precise definitions to help clinicians evaluate and treat chronic pain patients. *Journal of Pain & Palliative Care Pharmacotherapy,* **17** (1), 15–29.

Katz, NP, Sherburne, S, Beach, M, et al. (2003) Behavioral monitoring and urine toxicology testing in patients receiving long-term opioid therapy. *Anesth Analg,* **97**, 1097–1102.

Kripalani, S, Yao, X & Haynes, RB (2007) Interventions to enhance medication adherence in chronic medical conditions: a systematic review. *Arch Intern Med.,* **167** (6), 540–550.

CHAPTER 12

Pain in Children

Suellen M Walker

University College London, Institute of Child Health and Great Ormond Street Hospital for Children, London, UK

OVERVIEW

- Treatment of pain in children should be guided by pain assessment, using measurement tools that are appropriate to the age and developmental stage of the child

- Analgesics can be given safely to children, but the doses required for analgesia and the susceptibility to side effects can vary with age

- Even relatively brief medical procedures can be a significant source of pain and distress for children, and both pharmacological and non-pharmacological treatment strategies should be considered

- As a high proportion of paediatric surgery is performed on a day-case basis and parents will be responsible for continuing pain management, adequate instruction about expected pain, pain assessment and analgesic dosing is required prior to discharge

---

Pain assessment

Observer pain scores

In infants and preverbal children, assessment is dependent on observer evaluation of physiological and/or behavioural responses (Figure 12.1). As physiological measures are influenced by inter-current illness and drug treatments, they are more often used in combination with behavioural responses in composite measurement tools (e.g. COMFORT is recommended for infants and children in intensive care; Table 12.1). The context of testing is important, as infant responses may overlap with other states of distress (e.g. hunger and fatigue). The FLACC scale scores five behaviours and has been validated for both acute procedural and postoperative pain (Table 12.2). Specific tools are also available for children with cognitive impairment (e.g. NCCPC, Non-Communicating Children's Pain Checklist).

Self-report

Children aged 4–5 years can use a graded pictorial scale (e.g. faces scales) but they are more likely to choose the extremes of the

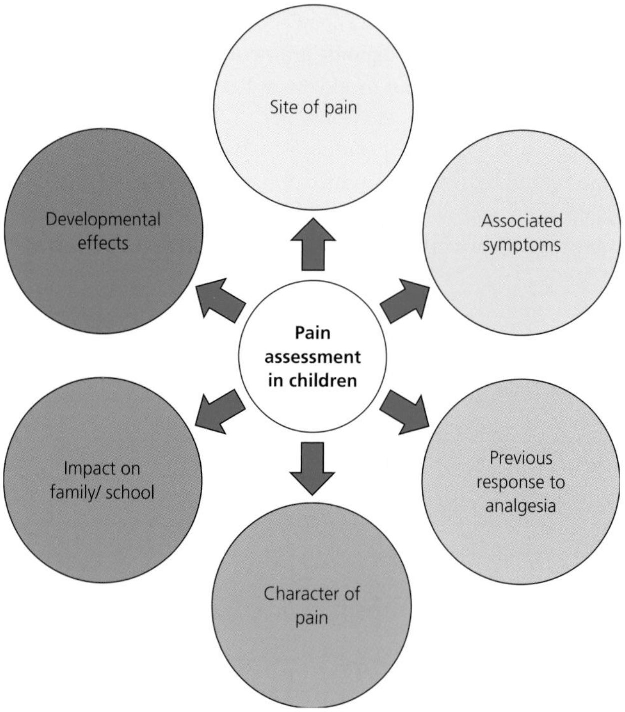

Figure 12.1 Assessment of pain in children requires assessment of many similar domains to those in adults, but may pose particular challenges, especially in non-specialist settings. A large number of measurement tools have been developed for children of different ages and for different clinical settings. Data from The Royal College of Nursing.

scale. In scales anchored with smiling or tearful faces, pain may be confused with other emotional states such as happiness/sadness or anxiety. In research trials, the Faces Pain Scale-Revised has been recommended for acute procedure-related, post-operative and disease-related pain for children aged 4–12 years. In clinical practice, standardised use of the same tool throughout an institution may be more important than which tool is chosen. Between seven and ten years children develop skills with measurement and can differentiate between the intervals on a scale and score their pain (e.g. 0–10 on a visual analogue scale). It is often not until 10–12 years of age that children can discriminate clearly between the sensory intensity and the affective emotional components of pain and report them independently.

ABC of Pain, First edition. Edited by Lesley A Colvin and Marie Fallon.
© 2012 Blackwell Publishing Ltd. Published 2012 by Blackwell Publishing Ltd.

Table 12.1 COMFORT pain scale.*

Category	Scoring				
	1	2	3	4	5
Alertness	Deeply asleep	Lightly asleep	Drowsy	Fully awake and alert	Hyperalert
Calmness	Calm	Slightly anxious	Anxious	Very anxious	Panicky
Respiratory response	No coughing or spontaneous respiration	Spontaneous respiration with little or no response to ventilation	Occasional cough or resistance to ventilator	Actively breathes against ventilator or coughs	Fights ventilator, coughing or choking
Physical movement	No movement	Occasional, slight movement	Frequent, slight movements	Vigorous movement of extremities	Vigorous movements including torso and head
Facial tone	Facial muscles relaxed	No facial muscle tension	Tension in some facial muscles	Tension throughout facial muscles	Facial muscles contorted and grimacing
Muscle tone	Totally relaxed	Reduced tone	Normal tone	Increased tone and flexion of fingers and toes	Extreme muscle rigidity
Blood pressure	BP below baseline	BP at baseline	Infrequent elevations 15% above baseline	Frequent elevations >15% above baseline	Sustained elevation >15% above baseline
Heart rate	HR below baseline	HR at baseline	Infrequent elevations 15% above baseline	Frequent elevations >15% above baseline	Sustained elevation >15% above baseline

* Ambuel, B, Hamlett, KW, Marx, CM, et al. (1992) Assessing distress in pediatric intensive care environments: the COMFORT scale. *J. Pediatr Psychol*, **17**, 95–109.

Table 12.2 FLACC pain scale.*

Category	Scoring		
	0	1	2
Face	No particular expression or smile	Occasional grimace or frown, withdrawn, disinterested	Frequent to constant quivering chin, clenched jaw
Legs	Normal position or relaxed	Uneasy, restless, tense	Kicking, or legs drawn up
Activity	Lying quietly, normal position, moves easily	Squirming, shifting back and forth, tense	Arched, rigid or jerking
Cry	No cry (awake or asleep)	Moans or whimpers; occasional complaint	Crying steadily, screams or sobs, frequent complaints
Consolability	Content, relaxed	Reassured by occasional touching, hugging or being talked to; distractable	Difficult to console or comfort

* Merkel, SI, Voepel-Lewis, T, Shayevitz, JR and Malviya, S (1997) The FLACC: a behavioral scale for scoring postoperative pain in young children. *Pediatr Nurs*, **23**, 293–297.

Analgesia

The efficacy and dose requirement for analgesics can vary significantly with age and depend on multiple factors (Figure 12.2). Clinical pharmacokinetic studies have established dose protocols that minimise side effects or toxicity. Pharmacodynamic effects also need to be considered, as age-related changes in receptor distribution and function may influence analgesic efficacy. For further details of analgesic use and dose recommendations see Further Reading and the British National Formulary for Children (http://bnfc.org/bnfc/).

Opioids

Morphine can be given safely at all ages with appropriate dosing and monitoring. As individual requirements vary and there is no clear correlation between plasma morphine concentration and analgesia, doses need to be titrated against effect. In neonates and infants this is often achieved by intravenous infusion with nurse-administered additional boluses as required. With adequate instruction, children aged over 5–6 years can self-administer doses via a patient controlled (PCA) device.

The analgesic effect of codeine is wholly or mainly reliant on metabolism to morphine by the cytochrome P450 enzyme

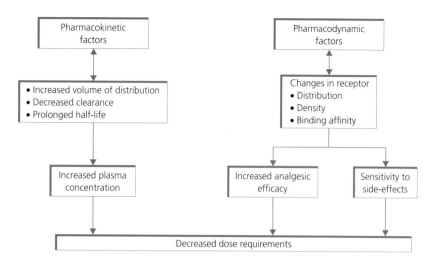

Figure 12.2 Morphine dose requirements in early life. Multiple factors influence dose requirements for analgesics in early life. Changes in the pharmacokinetic handling of morphine result in higher plasma concentrations and a prolonged duration of action following single doses; to compensate, dose intervals need to be increased and infusion rates decreased. In addition, changes in the body's response to morphine (i.e. pharmacodynamic effects) are altered by changes in receptor distribution and function, and as a result analgesic efficacy is achieved by lower plasma concentrations.

CYP2D6. In children with a genetically determined decrease in enzyme activity (up to 40% of a UK population), the efficacy of codeine is reduced. In addition, there is reduced CYP2D6 activity in neonates and infants.

Non-steroidal anti-inflammatory drugs (NSAIDs) and paracetamol

Non-steroidal anti-inflammatory drugs (NSAIDs) and paracetamol are effective for mild to moderate pain, and are often given in conjunction with opioids or local anaesthetic techniques for more severe pain. It has been estimated that 1:1000 asthmatics are susceptible to bronchospasm following NSAIDs, and although best avoided during acute asthma many children will tolerate NSAIDs without any increase in wheeze. NSAIDs decrease platelet function and may increase the risk of bleeding. Although an increased incidence of re-operation for bleeding has been associated with perioperative NSAID use and tonsillectomy, the risk appears low with diclofenac and ibuprofen in children. Higher doses of paracetamol are required for analgesia than for anti-pyretic effects. As the clearance of paracetamol is reduced in younger patients, the dose interval should be increased and the maximum daily dose reduced (Table 12.3).

Local anaesthesia

Topical local anaesthetic preparations provide effective analgesia for a range of procedural interventions in children. Amethocaine (e.g. Ametop) has a faster onset than the prilocaine–lidocaine mixture (EMLA) (20–30 minutes versus 50–60 minutes), but both require application under an occlusive dressing. Local anaesthetic techniques, such as wound infiltration, peripheral nerve blocks, caudal injections and epidural infusions, are frequently employed for perioperative analgesia in children of all ages. As excessive doses of local anaesthetic can produce cardiovascular and central nervous system toxicity, including arrhythmias and convulsions, maximum recommended doses should be calculated prior to injection (Table 12.4).

Procedural pain

Diagnostic and therapeutic procedural interventions (e.g. blood sampling, lumbar puncture, suture lacerations) can be a significant source of pain and distress for children. Effective management requires:

i *an analgesic plan*. This should be suited to the type of procedure and the child's preferences. An adequate dose of analgesic should be given at the appropriate time (e.g. topical LA requires 30–60 min to be effective depending on the preparation). Specialised techniques such as inhalation of nitrous oxide can be very effective if appropriate staffing and facilities are available. Some children may require general anaesthesia.

ii *non-pharmacological measures* may be sufficient for some procedures and should be used in combination with pharmacological treatments whenever possible. Breast feeding, sucking on pacifiers and sucrose solutions reduce behavioural responses to brief procedures in neonates. In older children, techniques such as distraction, relaxation, guided imagery and hypnosis can reduce pain and distress.

iii *environmental factors*. Parental presence and a quiet 'child friendly' room may minimise distress.

iv *procedure modification*. Tissue adhesives may be preferable to suturing for minor lacerations. Prior application of topical local anaesthetic or addition of bicarbonate to the solution reduces the pain of local anaesthetic injection. Some immunisation formulations are less painful on injection, and deeper intramuscular administration produces less local reaction afterwards than subcutaneous injection. If blood sampling is required, topical local anaesthetic is more effective for venepuncture than for heel lance.

Post-operative pain

A plan for perioperative analgesia should be discussed with the parent or guardian and the child, and be appropriate for the child's age, type of procedure and the clinical setting. In hospital, care is often coordinated by an acute pain service, with frequent assessment

Table 12.3 Suggested doses for NSAIDs and paracetamol.

	Age	Dose (mg/kg)	Interval (hours)	Maximum daily) dose (mg/kg/day)	Duration at maximum dose (hours)
Paracetamol	neonate	10–15	8–12	30	48
	1–6 months	15	6–8	60	48
	>6 months	15	4	90	72
Ibuprofen	>3 months	5–10	6–8	40	–
Diclofenac	>6 months	1	8	3	–

Table 12.4 Local anaesthetic preparations and suggested doses.

TOPICAL	Preparation	Onset	Duration[2]	Dose
EMLA[1]	2.5% lidocaine + 2.5% prilocaine	60 min	1–2 h (after removal)	3–12 months: 2 g 1–5 years: 10 g 6–11 years: 20 g
Ametop[1]	4% amethocaine	30 min	4–6 h (after removal)	0.5 g
Lidocaine	1% = 10 mg/ml 2% = 20 mg/ml 1% with epinephrine		30 min to 2 h 2–4 h	3 mg/kg 7 mg/kg
Bupivacaine	0.25% = 2.5 mg/ml		4–6 h	2–2.5 mg/kg[3]
Ropivacaine[4]	0.2% = 2 mg/ml		4–6 h	2–2.5 mg/kg[3]
Levobupivacaine[4]	0.25% = 2.5 mg/ml 0.5% = 5 mg/ml		4–6 h	2–2.5 mg/kg[3]

[1]Not recommended in neonates but safe use has been documented if no intercurrent methaemagloniaemia or anaemia.
[2]After single topical application or wound infiltration.
[3]Lower dose in neonates.
[4]Ropivacaine and levobupivacaine are L-isomers with similar efficacy but reduced systemic toxicity compared to the racemic mixture of bupivacaine.

of pain control, monitoring and management of side effects. As in adult practice, a multimodal approach is used with different analgesics targeting multiple mechanisms. Non-pharmacological measures should also be considered to reduce pain and distress. Details of postoperative pain management are available in recent evidence-based guidelines (see Further reading).

As a large proportion of paediatric surgery is now performed as day case admissions, families require information about pain assessment and analgesic use following discharge. Parents may be reluctant to give medication for fear of side effects, and clear verbal (and ideally written) instructions on appropriate doses and time intervals for analgesics are required, in addition to details of the likely severity and duration of post-operative pain. If local anaesthetic techniques have been used, parents should be aware of the potential for increased pain when the block wears off. Significant levels of pain, behavioural disturbance, sleep disruption and altered activity can persist for 5–8 days following tonsillectomy, and regular administration of paracetamol and NSAIDs may be necessary throughout this period.

Chronic pain

Chronic pain in children requires recognition and appropriate management, as it can have: significant social and emotional consequences for the child and family; physical and psychological sequelae; and disability that may impact on overall health and school attendance. Management within a multidisciplinary chronic pain service incorporating medical management of analgesic interventions, physiotherapy and rehabilitation, and psychological assessment and management may be required.

Potential causes of chronic pain in children include:

i   *chronic recurrent pain syndromes* (e.g. headache, recurrent abdominal pain, limb pain). These can occur in up to 25% of children.
ii *medical illnesses.* Conditions such as juvenile rheumatoid arthritis, sickle cell disease and degenerative neurological diseases can be associated with significant levels of pain and disability. Treatment is generally directed at the underlying condition but symptomatic control of pain is often required.
iii *cancer.* The pattern of cancer-related pain in children differs from adults. Pain is often present at the time of diagnosis of haematological malignancies but often improves following cancer-related treatment. Solid tumours, such as neuroblastoma, are less common but are more likely to be associated with continuing pain. Pain related to treatment is a major problem for children with cancer, due to repeated procedural interventions (e.g. lumbar punctures and bone marrow aspirations) or secondary to side-effects of radiotherapy and chemotherapy (e.g. mucositis).

iv *neuropathic pain* is increasingly recognised in children and may be related to traumatic or surgical injury (e.g. phantom limb pain). Few controlled trials have been conducted in children with chronic pain and treatment tends to be based empirically on data from adults (e.g. use of tricyclic antidepressants and gabapentin). Nerve injury in early life (e.g. brachial plexus palsy at time of delivery) is much less likely to cause pain than injuries in older children. Complex Regional Pain Syndrome (CRPS) occurs in children with a peak incidence around 11 years of age, a higher incidence in girls, and in contrast to adults is more likely to involve the lower limb. Maintenance of weight bearing, physiotherapy and non-invasive techniques are the focus of therapy.

Further reading

Friedrichsdorf, SJ, Finney, D, Bergin, M, Stevens, M & Collins, JJ (2007) Breakthrough Pain in Children with Cancer. *J Pain Symptom Manage*, **34**, 209–216.

Howard, RF, Carter, B, Curry, J, Morton, N, Rivett, K, Rose, M, et al. (2008) Association of Paediatric Anaesthetists: Good Practice in Postoperative and Procedural Pain. *Pediatric Anesthesia*, **18** (Suppl. 1), 1–81. (http://www.apagbi.org.uk/sites/apagbi.org.uk/files/APA%20Guideline%20part%201.pdf)

Macintyre, PE, Schug, SA, Scott, DA, Visser, EJ & Walker, SM [APM:SE Working Group of the Australian and New Zealand College of Anaesthetists and Faculty of Pain Medicine] (2010). *Acute Pain Management: Scientific Evidence*, 3rd edn. Melbourne: ANZCA & FPM. (http://www.fpm.anzca.edu.au/resources/books-and-publications/publications-1/Acute%20Pain%20-%20final%20version.pdf)

Royal College of Nursing (2009) *Clinical practice guidelines: The recognition and assessment of acute pain in children*. London: Royal College of Nursing. (http://www.rcn.org.uk/development/practice/clinicalguidelines/pain)

Schechter, NL, Zempsky, WT, Cohen, LL, McGrath, PJ, McMurtry, CM & Bright, NS (2007) Pain reduction during pediatric immunizations: evidence-based review and recommendations. *Pediatrics*, **119** (5), e1184–1198.

Tomlinson, D, von Baeyer, CL, Stinson, JN & Sung, L (2010) A systematic review of faces scales for the self-report of pain intensity in children. *Pediatrics*, **126**, e1168–e1198.

CHAPTER 13

Pain in Older Adults

Debra K Weiner

Geriatric Research, Education and Clinical Center, VA Pittsburgh Healthcare System and University of Pittsburgh School of Medicine, Pittsburgh, PA, USA

OVERVIEW

- Pain in older adults should be managed aggressively because of its potential deleterious impact on mental, emotional, and physical function

- Pain is only one of many things that can contribute to disability in older adults (e.g. dementia, social isolation), thus its treatment should occur with these other factors in mind

- Each older adult's unique pain signature should be determined at the start of treatment so that the effectiveness of treatment can be determined

- Contributors to chronic pain in older adults are typically multiple

- A stepped care approach to treatment should be used, starting with modalities associated with the least potential systemic toxicity; all contributors to the pain syndrome must be targeted

---

Introduction

As the world increasingly greys, so too does the need for practitioners to gain competence in caring for older adults with a myriad of pain conditions. While many of these patients have suffered from pain for decades, others, because of the accumulation of degenerative pathology in their later years, are relative newcomers to pain. In either case, pain should never be considered normal and because older adults are not simply a chronologically older version of younger patients with pain, unique skills are needed to afford optimal treatment outcomes in these individuals.

This chapter focuses on chronic or persistent pain because of its greater clinical complexity and treatment challenges. Because aging in the absence of pain also may be associated with deterioration in each of these domains, aggressive treatment of chronic pain in older adults is especially important (Figure 13.1).

Evaluation

The key to optimising treatment outcomes lies in careful and comprehensive evaluation (Figure 13.2).

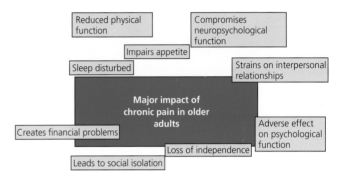

Figure 13.1 Multiple important functional domains that may be impacted by chronic pain.

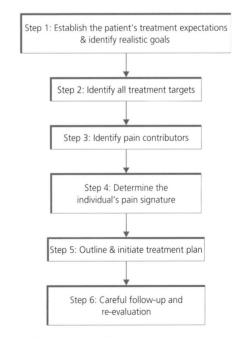

Figure 13.2 Pain evaluation in older adults.

Step 1: Establish the patient's treatment expectations

The first step in evaluation is to establish what the patient expects from treatment and to set realistic goals. If the patient's treatment expectations are unrealistic (e.g. a pain-free state), these must be

ABC of Pain, First edition. Edited by Lesley A Colvin and Marie Fallon.
© 2012 Blackwell Publishing Ltd. Published 2012 by Blackwell Publishing Ltd.

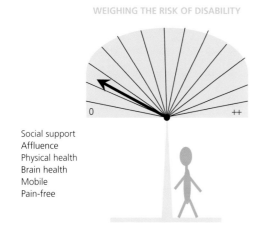

WEIGHING THE RISK OF DISABILITY

Social support
Affluence
Physical health
Brain health
Mobile
Pain-free

Figure 13.3 Factors contributing to a low risk of disability.

reconciled to avoid frustration on the part of both patient and practitioner. Depending upon the setting of care and the patient's cognitive status, involving the caregiver(s) may be critical at this stage.

Step 2: Identify all treatment targets

Once realistic treatment expectations and patient goals have been established, the next step is to explore the factors that need to be targeted to improve pain management. Chronic pain may be only one of multiple factors that increase the risk of disability and impair quality of life in older adults. For the older adult with good social support, financial resources, physical and emotional health, and who is independent in mobility and free of pain, the risk of disability is low (Figure 13.3).

For the individual who is socially isolated, indigent, burdened with multiple medical and psychological comorbidities, immobility and chronic pain, the risk of disability and poor quality of life is quite high (Figure 13.4). It is incumbent upon the practitioner, therefore, to prioritise and tailor chronic pain treatment according to the context in which it exists.

In the older adult with severe dementia, for example, it may be that the dementia itself is the main contributor to impaired function and overall distress. While such a patient's pain requires

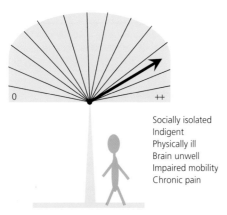

Socially isolated
Indigent
Physically ill
Brain unwell
Impaired mobility
Chronic pain

Figure 13.4 High risk of disability.

treatment, the approach to pain treatment may be very different as compared with the treatment of chronic pain in a cognitively intact, highly functioning individual, as illustrated by the case history example in Box 13.1.

Box 13.1 **Case history: Pain management in the elderly**

82-year old woman:

Pain history: two years of low back pain after retiring; intensity increased by prolonged standing or walking; improved by local application of heat. No associated fever, chills, weight loss, paresthesias, lower extremity weakness, or change in function of her bowels or bladder. She denied nocturnal symptoms.

Social history: had been working full time but retired due to company downsizing two years ago; lived alone – harder to do housework; frequent near-falls; passive suicidal ideations, and fear of going on the bus alone, so spending more time at home alone.

Medication: gabapentin, oxycodone CR, celecoxib, tramadol, acetaminophen, olanzapine, escitalopram, and lorazepam.

Examination: very impaired righting reflexes (i.e. inability to right herself in response to a gentle backwards tug at the waist) and performance on the clock drawing test (consistent with dementia); marked kyphoscoliosis, and tenderness on palpation of the right sacroiliac joint, tensor fascia lata (TFL) and erector spinae. Strength testing was limited by extreme guarding behaviour.

Management: admitted to a nursing home for detoxification; all medications were discontinued except regularly scheduled acetaminophen and prn tramadol; physical therapy for gait training and for treatment of her TFL myofascial pain and dysfunction. Her balance and cognitive function improved markedly and her pain complaints became infrequent. Assisted living facility placement was recommended–social isolation and mild dementia were felt to have significantly contributed to her pain complaints–but the patient and her family refused.

Outcome: Within 24 hours of discharge, the patient's pain complaints escalated–frequent calls asking for more pain medication: the physician remained firm in her conviction that the patient's social situation was driving her pain behaviour so the analgesic regimen was not changed. Another pain provider escalated her pain medication regimen (including a failed morphine pump trial). Ultimately the patient was admitted to an assisted living facility, where she did well.

Learning points from this case:

- Social isolation and associated fear were the main factors driving the patient's disability, not her pain.
- Attention to these factors held the key to her improvement.
- Focus on treatment of her pain to the exclusion of these other factors exposed the patient to unnecessary morbidity risk and inappropriate use of healthcare resources.

Step 3: Identify the pain contributors

If treatment of pain per se is a primary treatment target, the next step is to identify the factors that may be contributing to the pain. Causes of pain in older adults broadly can be divided, as with younger patients, into nociceptive and neuropathic causes. Common causes

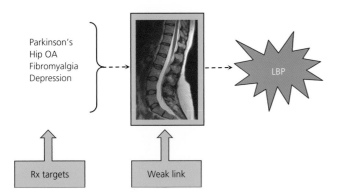

Parkinson's
Hip OA
Fibromyalgia
Depression

LBP

Rx targets

Weak link

Figure 13.5 Degenerative pathology of the lumbar spine is only one factor that contributes to pain and disability in the older adult with low back pain.

of nociceptive pain include osteoarthritis, myofascial pain and low back pain (LBP). Typically multiple factors contribute to myofascial pain and low back pain. For example, in the older adult with chronic low back pain, underlying pathologies that often co-exist are lumbar spinal stenosis, sacroiliac joint syndrome related to degenerative scoliosis and/or hip osteoarthritis, myofascial dysfunction and fibromyalgia. Effective treatment in such an individual, therefore, requires attention to each of these conditions. The diagnosis of these contributors relies almost exclusively on a careful history and physical examination. No laboratory testing is required, with the exception of hip osteoarthritis, the diagnosis of which is confirmed with a plain radiograph. X-rays and MRIs of the lumbar spine are not needed in the majority of older adults with chronic low back pain. Most older adults without pain have degenerative disc and facet disease and an estimated one in five without neurogenic claudication has MRI evidence of lumbar spinal stenosis. Thus, degenerative pathology should be thought of as the weak link rather than the sole treatment target in these individuals (Figure 13.5).

Important causes of neuropathic pain to consider in older adults include diabetic peripheral neuropathy, paraneoplastic neuropathy and post-herpetic neuralgia.

Other possible pain contributors include: chronic widespread pain, which can have features of both nociceptive pain and neuropathic pain, is also common in older adults; fibromyalgia syndrome (FMS) is common in this age group. Key disorders to consider in the differential diagnosis are shown in Box 13.2.

Box 13.2 **Differential diagnosis of widespread pain in older adults**

Fibromyalgia Syndrome
Generalised Osteoarthritis
Pseudogout
Gout
Rheumatoid Arthritis
Systemic Lupus Erythematosus
Polymyalgia Rheumatica/Temporal Arteritis
Vitamin D Deficiency
Hypothyroidism
Adverse Drug Reactions (e.g. statins)

Key co-morbidities that require treatment in order to optimise pain control (e.g. depression or anxiety) or that may enhance risks associated with treatment (e.g. pre-existing mobility dysfunction and falls, history of delirium associated with opioids, dementia) must also be identified at this stage to facilitate a comprehensive treatment plan. Co-morbidities that the practitioner must screen in all older adults with chronic pain are listed in Box 13.3.

Box 13.3 **Key co-morbidities in the older adult**

Dementia
Depression
Anxiety
Social Isolation
Impaired Mobility Status and Falls Risk
Functional Dependence
Malnutrition

Step 4: Determine the 'pain signature'

In parallel with determining contributors to the patient's pain and before treatment is initiated, the individual's 'pain signature' must be determined. Pain may impact the older adult many ways, as listed in Table 13.1. Identifying the ways that pain affects each patient allows the practitioner to determine whether his or her treatment has truly helped.

Step 5: Outline a treatment plan

After the contributors to the patient's pain syndrome have been identified and their pain signature ascertained, a treatment plan should be outlined. A suggested stepped care approach for the treatment of nociceptive pain is shown in Figure 13.6. At the foundation of the treatment lies education that includes instruction in self-management techniques, a regular exercise programme with as much aerobic activity as possible, weight loss (especially for patients with degenerative disease of the lower back and lower extremities) and the use of assistive devices to facilitate mobility and for joint unloading. The remaining steps in the pyramid shown in Figure 13.6 represent progression from interventions associated with minimal potential risk to those associated with substantial potential risk. While injections are invasive, in this chapter they are considered relatively low risk as compared with the potential for adverse reactions associated with exposing the older adult to systemic medications. Especially for the patient with localised pain,

Table 13.1 The pain signature: possible elements.

Parameter	Possible manifestations
Behaviour	Agitation, withdrawal, aggressiveness
Mental Status	Increased confusion
Nutritional Status	Decreased appetite and weight loss
Mobility	Pacing, increased instability, weakness and more difficulty ambulating
Mood	Depression, anxiety, irritability

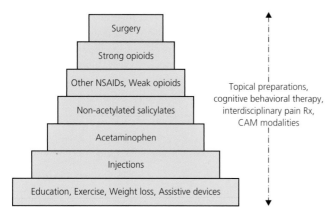

Figure 13.6 Stepped care approach to treatment of nociceptive pain. NSAID = non-steroidal anti-inflammatory drug, CAM = complementary and alternative medicine. Reprinted from *Pain in Older Persons*, IASP Press 2005, with permission from the International Association for the Study of Pain.

such as that associated with knee osteoarthritis, tendinitis, and myofascial pain, local injection procedures should be considered routinely as first line treatment.

The risks associated with the systemic medication classes shown in Figure 13.6 have been well documented. Non-steroidal anti-inflammatory medications have a number of associated risks, including renal impairment, cerebrovascular accidents, heart failure and gastrointestinal bleeding. Opioids may be associated with delirium, falls and hip fractures. It is important to recognise, however, that pain itself may be associated with delirium, thus the relative risks and benefits of opioids must be weighed carefully and the patient followed closely if a decision is made to initiate opioid therapy. Every effort should be made to optimise the patient's mobility and stability (e.g. prescription of an assistive device, referral to a physiotherapist) before opioids are prescribed, given their association with falls and hip fractures. This risk must be emphasised to the patient and their family.

Remember other co-morbidities

At all steps of treatment, treatment of other co-morbidities that contribute to pain and its effects on the patient must be pursued. Patients with anxiety, depression and/or poor coping skills will not improve to their full potential unless these conditions are treated aggressively.

Neuropathic pain

Medications for the treatment of neuropathic pain have been discussed elsewhere in this book (Chapter 6). Titration schedules in the elderly need to take account of relative sensitivity to centrally acting agents. Topical preparations, such as a lidocaine patch, the new 8% capsaicin patch or other compounded agents (e.g. ketamine or combination products), may be useful for the treatment of localised neuropathic pain, such as post-herpetic neuralgia or post-surgical neuropathic pain. It is important to recognise that since nerve

fibres course through musculature, myofascial dysfunction may be associated with neuropathic pain. In these cases, treatment directed toward the myofascial pathology (e.g. gentle stretching and strengthening, trigger point deactivation) may be associated with significant relief of neuropathic symptoms.

Chronic widespread pain

Treatment should be guided by the underlying cause (Table 13.1). Treatment of fibromyalgia syndrome (FMS) is reviewed elsewhere in this book (Chapter 4) and treatment of older adults with FMS should be guided by these pharmacological and non-pharmacological guidelines. Unfortunately, medications associated with strong efficacy evidence, such as cyclobenzaprine, amitriptyline and pregabalin, may be associated with sedation and other untoward side effects in older adults. If a tricyclic antidepressant is determined to be the most appropriate agent, one with low anticholinergic potential (e.g.desipramine, nortriptyline) should be chosen. Gabapentin is less potent than pregabalin and has not been approved for the treatment of FMS, but this author has successfully treated many older adults with FMS using low doses of this medication (e.g. 100 mg po four times daily, titrated by 100 mg per week to a total daily dose of 300–600 mg qd – bid).

Step 6: Follow-up and reassessment

After treatment has been initiated, careful follow-up must ensue to determine its impact, both beneficial and deleterious. The practitioner should refer back to the patient's pain signature as a frame of reference. One of the most important things for the practitioner to keep in mind is that chronic pain is a condition to be managed, not cured, thus continuing follow-up is critical.

Further reading

Camacho-Soto, A, Sowa, G & Weiner, DK (2011) Geriatric Pain. In: Benzon, H, Raja, S, Fishman, S, Liu, S & Cohen, SP (eds), *Essentials of Pain Medicine*, 3rd edn. Elsevier.

Finando, D & Finando, S (2005). *Trigger Point Therapy for Myofascial Pain – The Practice of Informed Touch*. Rochester, VT: Healing Arts Press.

Gibson, SJ & Weiner, DK (eds) (2005) *Pain in Older Persons, Progress in Pain Research and Management*, Vol. 35. Seattle, WA: IASP Press.

Karp, JF, Shega, JW, Morone, NE & Weiner, DK (2008) Advances in understanding the mechanisms and management of persistent pain in older adults. *British Journal of Anaesthesia*, **101** (1), 111–120.

Resnick, NM & Marcantonio, ER (1997) How should clinical care of the aged differ? *Lancet*, **350**, 1157–1158.

Shega, J, Emanuel, L, Vargish, L, Levine, SK, Bursch, H, Herr, K, *et al.* (2007) Pain in persons with dementia: complex, common, and challenging. *Journal of Pain*, **8** (5), 373–378.

Weiner, DK (2007) Office management of chronic pain in the elderly. *American Journal of Medicine*, **120**, 306–315.

Weiner, DK, Sakamoto, S, Perera, S & Breuer, P (2006) Chronic low back pain in older adults: prevalence, reliability, and validity of physical examination findings. *J Am GeriatrSoc*, **54**, 11–20.

CHAPTER 14

Pain in Pregnancy

George R Harrison

Department of Pain Management, Queen Elizabeth Hospital Birmingham, Birmingham, UK

OVERVIEW

- Pregnant women have to undergo enormous physical and physiological changes to cope with the rapid growth of an intra-abdominal tumour

- Musculoskeletal pain is very common but can often be managed with physiotherapy and acupuncture

- The acute abdomen in pregnancy is often difficult to diagnose, and newer magnetic imaging techniques can provide diagnostic information without putting the foetus at risk.

- Patients with pre-existing chronic pain need counselling before pregnancy to ensure they understand the implications that pregnancy will have upon the management of their pain

- In pregnancy the number of analgesics that are safe to use is restricted due to the risks of teratogenesis and post-partum developmental problems

---

Introduction

Pregnancy is a common physiological variation of the normal condition of women but is accompanied by various changes, physiological and pathological, which may be associated with severe pain, the inevitable one for most women being that of labour (not addressed here). However, it is important to be aware of the physiological changes in pregnancy, as they will help to explain some of the problems of pain that seem to be specific to pregnancy (Table 14.1). Many of these changes are necessary in response to the development of a rapidly growing intra-abdominal tumour, in particular there will be changes to the musculoskeletal system, augmented by hormonal changes. Alongside this there are changes to other organs and systems within the body, which will have an impact upon the pharmacokinetics and pharmacodynamics of drugs used in the treatment of pregnant women.

Pregnancy does not offer immunity to the normal vicissitudes of life, and therefore there are many causes of pain in pregnancy which are common to women in normal life (Figure 14.1).

Table 14.1 Physiological changes in pregnancy.

Gastro Intestinal Tract transit time	↑
Stomach acidity in 1ˢᵗ and 2ⁿᵈ Trimesters	↓
Gastric pH	↑
Circulating blood volume	↑
Cardiac output	↑
Renal outflow	↑
Creatinine clearance	↑
Body water	↑

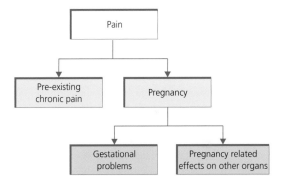

Figure 14.1 Factors leading to pain and discomfort during pregnancy. When there is pre-existing chronic pain, management of these patients may become much more complex, as their change of condition may radically altered the clinical situation.

Musculoskeletal problems

The development of an intra-abdominal mass will give rise to postural changes secondary to the shift in the centre of gravity of the body, with alterations of the spinal curves, possibly increasing the lumbar lordosis and, thereby, increasing the strain on the zygapophyseal joints. The muscles are also affected, the rectus abdominis muscles being lengthened, along with divarification or diastasis of the muscles. The oblique muscles will be changed not only in length but also the direction of action will be changed. Finally, there is often weakness or poor function of the gluteal muscles, which are important in postural maintenance. The changes in the joints of the lumbar spine and the pelvis are generally secondary to the hormonal changes of pregnancy, in particular the increase in relaxin levels, which has an effect upon the extensibility

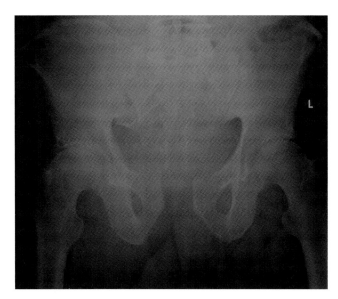

Figure 14.2 Diastalsis of the pubic symphysis is not uncommon in pregnancy and can lead to considerable pain and disability, with some women developing continuing problems after delivery.

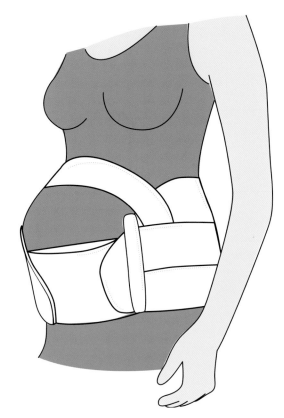

Figure 14.3 Pelvic belts may help to support the pelvis and sacroiliac joints.

of connective tissue. This will have a major impact upon the joints of the pelvis, particularly the sacroiliac joints and the pubic symphysis, notably with diastasis of the pubic ramus, but also with the forward rotation of the innominate bones associated with a counternutation (backward movement) of the sacrum, the end result of which is pelvic instability.

The prevalence of low back and pelvic pain in pregnancy (LBPP) is reported as 72%. This includes simple low back pain, but also isolated sacroiliac joint pain, pain from the symphysis pubis or a combination of all three (Figure 14.2). The predisposing factors are parity, previous LBPP, body mass index and hypermobility.

Treatment has been through physiotherapy, with various exercise regimes, but it has been shown that stabilising exercises are beneficial, and there is an increasing volume of evidence to demonstrate that acupuncture is a safe and highly effective method of improving pain and function. There is no evidence for the use of Transcutaneous Electrical Nerve Stimulation (TENS) machines, outside of labour, in pregnancy, although TENS machines have been used as long as the electrodes are not positioned directly over the abdomen (further information is given in Chapter 18). The use of pelvic belts has been advised, as they can stabilise the sacroiliac joints (Figure 14.3). Finally, there may be problems with the hip joint in pregnancy, namely idiopathic transient osteoporosis of the hip. This is a rare idiopathic disorder presenting with severe hip pain, which is normally self-limiting, resolving spontaneously in 6–24 months post-partum, but the use of agents to prevent the resorption of bone may reduce the duration of symptoms.

Gestational problems

Pregnancy itself can give rise to painful conditions starting in the first trimester (Figure 14.4). Miscarriage may be associated with pain with a reported incidence of up to 25% of recognised pregnancies. Ectopic pregnancy occurs in 1–2% of pregnancies with the

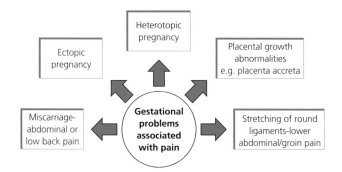

Figure 14.4 Painful conditions related to the pregnancy itself, which may start in the first trimester.

gestation sac present outside the body of the uterus. The presentation is frequently that of abdominal pain with a short history of amenorrhoea, and would normally be diagnosed with ultrasound. Surgical treatment is necessary. Heterotropic pregnancy is the presence of an ectopic pregnancy alongside a normal pregnancy, which will again present with acute abdominal pain. Surgical removal of the ectopic pregnancy is the treatment. Abnormalities of placental growth, such as placenta percreta, may present with pain, as may abruption of the placenta, which is associated with pain in about 50% of cases. Finally, the growth of the uterus will stretch the round ligament of the uterus, which gives rise to an intermittent pain, often in the lower abdomen, frequently extending into the groin.

Reproductive organs

Pain may arise from the ovaries secondary to torsion, or tumours, which can be either physiological, benign or malignant. The uterus too is at risk of torsion, defined as rotation of more than 45 degrees in the long axis of the uterus, occurring mainly in the third trimester. Uterine infection may be associated with pelvic pain, as will rupture of the uterus, although these are relatively uncommon. The more common problem is fibroids, which may grow in size during pregnancy and undergo degeneration.

Renal tract

As a result of pressure of the growing uterus on the ureter, hydronephrosis can occur, and is common in pregnancy, but infrequently symptomatic (0.2% pregnancies). Secondary symptoms may include renal colic, pyelonephritis, cystitis and renal abscesses. Generally, conservative treatment is sufficient but ureteric stenting may be required in recalcitrant cases.

Other abdominal viscera

All of the abdominal contents are at risk of developing pathological changes at any time, but in pregnancy the diagnosis may be less obvious due to the presence of the enlarged uterus. Anxiety about operating on pregnant women, with a putative attendant risk of miscarriage, may influence decision making. The presentation is frequently of an acute abdomen and diagnosis is potentially difficult, but with the use of MRI scanning diagnosis can be made successfully which can then inform the future management effectively (Table 14.2).

Pregnancy is a hypercoagulable state, with thrombo-embolic phenomena accounting for 2% of maternal deaths. Although the majority of cases will be associated with deep vein thrombosis of the peripheral circulation, there are reports of intra-abdominal thrombosis which can affect a variety of vessels. Those reported tend to be generally the larger vessels such as the inferior vena cava and iliac veins, although ovarian vein thrombosis is recognised. These may present as an acute abdomen, although inferior vena cava thrombosis has been known to present with sciatica.

Chronic pain and pregnancy

The management of the patient who has chronic pain, when pregnant, is a challenge to both the obstetrician and the pain clinician, especially when the pain is present before conception. In this circumstance counselling should be undertaken early, as there are issues that need to be considered by the patient, relating to both the management of the pain in pregnancy as well as the implications of having a child upon the future management of their condition, especially when this is a musculoskeletal problem. In the author's practice it has been found that even patients who are not so physically disabled by their condition find that parenthood adds new complications to their pain management.

Medication during pregnancy

Patients with chronic pain are often on a cocktail of drugs which they find necessary to help manage their pain. If they are determined to become pregnant, they have to realise that the number of drugs which are safe to use in pregnancy is limited, which may require them to alter or even cease using medication during their pregnancy. Also, some drugs may have to be stopped prior to conception if they wish to have the best chance of a successful pregnancy, specifically anti-inflammatory drugs, which are believed to increase the risk of spontaneous miscarriage by up to 100%.

Inflammatory or nociceptive pain

Nociceptive and inflammatory pain syndromes would generally respond to anti-inflammatory drugs and opioids. There are problems with anti-inflammatory drugs, as described above, but the evidence suggests that paracetamol is safe. Of all the opioids, morphine is the one drug that has been used for many years and there has not been any evidence of teratogenicity associated with its use. There is concern over the neonatal abstinence syndrome that occurs to the foetus after birth due to opiate withdrawal (Figure 14.5). This is reported particularly in women who have been taking the drug recreationally, but it is not clear if it is such a major problem in women who have been taking the drug for pain management. It is also worth noting that on the odd occasion when there is a specific pregnancy related pain problem which requires morphine to manage it, it is often found that there is no problem in withdrawing morphine once the need for it has gone. It would be preferable

Table 14.2 Causes of acute abdomen by organ.

Bowel	Intussusception
	Volvulus
	Appendicitis
Liver	Infarction
Gall Bladder	Acute cholecystitis
Pancreas	Pancreatitis
Spleen	Torsion
	Infarction
Adrenal gland	Haemorrhage
	Phaeochromocytoma

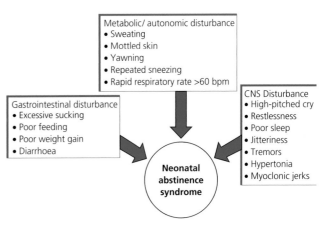

Figure 14.5 Some of the features that may be associated with Neonatal Abstinence Syndrome.

Table 14.3 Stigmata of foetal anticonvulsant syndrome.

–Speech delays
–Joint laxity
–Glue ear
–Facial dysmorphology
–Myopia
–Autism
–Hyperactivity

Table 14.4 Rate of major malformations with anti-epileptic drugs.

Drug	Malformation rate (%)
Phenobarbital	12
Valproate	5.9–8.6
Carbamazepine	2.3
Lamotrigine	1.8–2.1
Gabapentin	unknown, but one study showed no major malformation in babies of 11 mothers taking the drug in the first trimester. There is no evidence for Pregabalin in the literature

to manage such pain types with morphine, as there is not enough evidence to show that other opioids are safe, particularly the newer synthetic agents.

Neuropathic pain

Neuropathic pain is a bigger problem, as the drugs used to treat this are either antidepressants or anti-epileptic drugs (Chapter 6). The tricyclic antidepressants are not associated with teratogenesis, nor are they associated with developmental problems in the post-natal period. There is some evidence to support the development of complications after the use of SSRIs. Anti-epileptic drugs (AEDs) are different in that there is evidence to show that they can give rise to a specific syndrome (Table 14.3) as well as being teratogenic. The bulk of these data comes from the drug registers that are used to monitor these events (Table 14.4). There is little evidence available yet on the newer drugs specifically licensed for neuropathic pain, although the small series currently available look promising.

Further Reading

Birchard, KR, Brown, MA, Hyslop, WB, Firat, Z & Semelka, RC (2005) MRI of acute abdominal and pelvic pain in pregnant patients. *Am J Roentgenol*, **184**, 452–458

Elden, H, Ladfors, L, Olsen, MF, Ostgaard, HC & Hagberg, H (2005) Effects of acupuncture and stabilising exercises as adjunct to standard treatment in pregnant women with pelvic girdle pain: randomised single blind controlled trial. *BMJ*, **331**, 49–50

Fainaru, O, Almog, B, Gamzu, R, Lessing, JB & Kupferminc, M (2002) The management of symptomatic hydronephrosis in pregnancy. *BJOG*, **109**, 1385–1387

Kilpatrick, CC & Monga, M (2007) Approach to the acute abdomen in pregnancy. *Obstet Gynecol Clin North Am*, **34** (3), 389–402.

Lucas, S (2009) Medication use in the treatment of migraine during pregnancy and lactation. *Curr Pain Headache Rep*, **13**, 392–398.

Powrie, RO, Greene, MF & Camann, W (eds) (2010) *de Sweit's Medical disorders in obstetric practice*. John Wiley & Sons Ltd.

CHAPTER 15

Psychological Aspects of Chronic Pain

David Gillanders

University of Edinburgh/Lothian Chronic Pain Service, School of Health in Social Science, Edinburgh, UK

OVERVIEW

- Understanding psychological factors in pain is vital to helping chronic pain patients
- There is no good evidence for the psychogenic causation of pain
- Psychological accounts which emphasise the behavioural, cognitive and emotional consequences of pain and the impacts of these on pain itself have been more influential and more useful
- Psychologically-based treatments that target these processes have good evidence of their efficacy
- All health professionals can significantly influence a patients' healthcare trajectory by influencing their beliefs and appraisals of pain and its meaning

Introduction

People who experience chronic pain not only have symptoms such as pain, they also experience routinely other symptoms that may bring with them a multitude of other problems (Figure 15.1). In addition to understanding the symptoms and physiological mechanisms of chronic pain, clinicians must also develop an appreciation of the psychological consequences of developing a persistent pain problem.

Early involvement of psychology in pain management

Early multidisciplinary approaches to chronic pain looked to psychology to provide explanations for the development of pain in persons whose symptoms were unexplained medically. The psychology of the time was influenced heavily by psychoanalytic understandings, which took pain to be an expression of an underlying unconscious conflict. As such, the notion of pain as either organic or 'psychogenic' has become widespread. The evidence now suggests overwhelmingly that such a distinction is neither accurate scientifically nor helpful therapeutically. Whilst there are correlational studies that show an association between early life

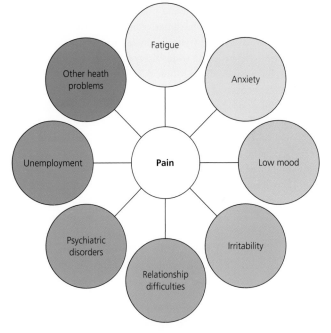

Figure 15.1 Other features commonly associated with pain.

trauma and certain types of pain, such as pelvic pain, there is no convincing evidence that chronic pain arises from a psychogenic causation. Whatever the reason why an individual's pain persists, psychology is much more useful in explaining how an individual responds to pain and how their behavioural, cognitive and emotional responses influence subsequently both their pain condition and their journey through the healthcare system.

Early work in the field of understanding pain began in earnest with the work of Wilbert Fordyce. He applied the behavioural principles of operant conditioning to explain how certain behaviours (grimacing, complaining of pain, resting) could be shaped by the responses of the pain patient's significant others. Fordyce reasoned that with repeated shaping of pain responses and reinforcement from others in the form of attention, reduced role burden and so on, the pain response itself became 'learned behaviour'. Early behaviour analysts used these principles to design behavioural treatments for chronic pain patients that reduced significant other's responding to maladaptive behaviours, whilst simultaneously increased responding to active behaviours. In addition, behavioural treatment involves establishing collaboratively a series of graded goals and helping the pain sufferer to work towards achieving these goals, step by step.

Cognitive behavioural therapy in pain management

In the 1960s and 1970s the development of computing led to a popularity of cognitive psychology, which attempts to model the processes of thinking, memory, judgement and attention (Figure 15.2). Cognitive psychology and behavioural psychology were blended in the Cognitive Behavioural Therapy (CBT) tradition. CBT was first applied successfully in randomised controlled trials to the treatment of major depressive disorder. CBT is now by far the most widely endorsed and practiced form of psychological therapy in the world and it has amassed an impressive evidence base of randomised controlled trials and meta-analyses, demonstrating its effectiveness in treating a wide variety of psychiatric and physical health problems, including chronic pain.

The effectiveness of CBT for chronic pain stems from our understanding of the behavioural, cognitive and emotional consequences of persistent pain, and the consequences of these psychological responses on pain. These factors have been derived from basic and clinical research in the psychology of pain. The most influential understandings of chronic pain have come from The Fear–Avoidance Model (originally proposed by Vlaeyen and co-workers in 1995) (Figure 15.3), catastrophising-based accounts (Sullivan *et al.*, 1995), accounts related to attribution and appraisal (such as from Crombez, and Vlaeyen) (Crombez *et al.*, 1999; Vlaeyen & Linton, 2000) and, more recently, accounts based on Acceptance and Commitment Therapy (as developed by McCracken and co-workers) (McCracken & Eccleston, 2003).

The Fear–Avoidance Model of chronic pain

The Fear–Avoidance Model (Figure 15.4) provides a basis for understanding why the degree of disability varies so much among

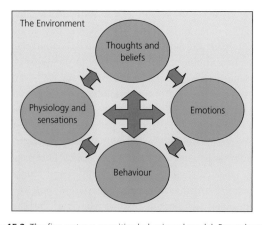

Figure 15.2 The five systems cognitive behavioural model. Reproduced with permission from Padesky, C.A. & Mooney, K.A. (1990). Clinical tip: Presenting the cognitive model to clients. *International Cognitive Therapy Newsletter*, **6**, 13–14. (available from www.padesky.com/clinicalcorner.htm)

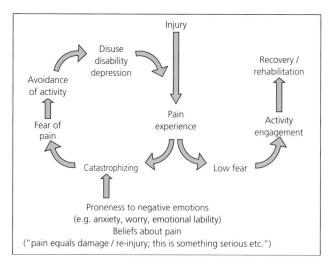

Figure 15.3 The Fear–Avoidance Model. (Adapted from Leeuw *et al.*, 2007).

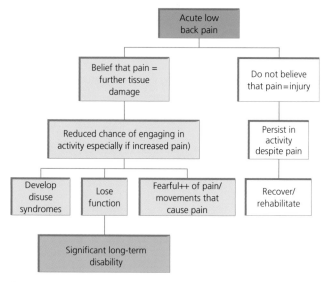

Figure 15.4 The Fear–Avoidance Model of chronic pain predicts that the primary difference between individuals who recover or rehabilitate successfully from an experience of acute low back pain and those do not, are the beliefs they hold and the behaviours that flow from these beliefs.

individuals and allows this to be addressed. This may be seen in those patients who believe: 'Maybe this pain means I am making myself worse'.

As fear of pain develops, the individual develops an attentional focus on pain, increased arousal, reduced activity and further catastrophic misinterpretation of pain sensations as signalling damage. As a result of reduced activity and a seemingly inescapable pain problem, individuals will be more likely to develop mood problems, which alter the threshold at which pain sensations will be perceived and responded to.

There is now significant evidence for each of the basic elements of the Fear–Avoidance Model in chronic low back pain. There is also evidence of pain-related beliefs, fear of pain and avoidance of pain being predictive of the development of low back pain disability, independent of pain intensity.

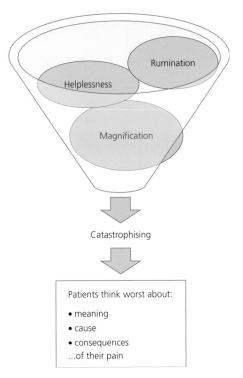

Figure 15.5 The concept of catastrophising is referred to as an exaggerated mental set of the cognitive aspects of pain related fear. As a result of this engagement of cognitive resources towards the pain, its disruptive effects on mood and activity are greatly increased. (Sullivan *et al.*, 2004).

Pain catastrophising

An important element of the Fear–Avoidance Model is catastrophic misinterpretation of pain sensations (Figure 15.5). Catastrophising can be measured readily using standardised self-report questionnaires and is thought to be a relatively stable dispositional trait. It has been shown to correlate highly with most important indices of functioning, including pain intensity, disability, distress, mood problems, quality of life, observable pain behaviour, spousal responding and activity avoidance. In addition, several prospective studies have demonstrated associations between initial levels of catastrophising and subsequent experiences of pain after surgery, pain during a painful procedure and in long-term adjustment to lower limb amputation.

Appraisal-based models

Both the Fear–Avoidance Model and the catastrophising account of pain responding contain significant elements of appraisals; people's interpretation of situations, their sensations, the world and themselves. Appraisal-based models have been influential in other medical conditions and are now being applied to the study of chronic pain. One example of these is the 'Common Sense Self-Regulatory Model' of Howard Leventhal. In the common sense model, individuals make appraisals of the meaning of their symptoms along the dimensions shown in Table 15.1.

Individuals label the identity of their medical condition according to the signs and symptoms associated with it, they appraise the consequences and timeline of their condition and whether cure

Table 15.1 Appraisal dimensions in the Common Sense Self-Regulatory Model.

• Identity	the signs and symptoms of this illness and the name given to it
• Timeline	whether this illness will last a long time or a short time
• Cause	attributions about the cause of the illness, e.g. genes, environment, stress, own behaviour, other's influence
• Consequences	the effects of having this illness on activity, employment, financial stability, relationships, sense of identity
• Cure/Controllability	the degree to which a cure is expected or the degree to which the illness and its symptoms can be controlled
• Emotional representations	the degree to which the illness effects emotions, e.g. 'My illness makes me angry' or 'My illness makes me sad'

Adapted from Leventhal *et al.* (1992).

is possible. In addition, people make emotional appraisals about their condition, for example that 'Being in pain makes me angry'. These appraisals influence an individual's use of coping strategies, emotional responses and subsequent behaviour.

Impact of pain on identity

A further addition to appraisal based models is the work by Morley and colleagues on pain and identity (Table 15.2). These authors

Table 15.2 Interruption, interference and identity.

	Brief description	Treatments focused at this level
Interruption	The impact of pain on moment-to-moment attention and behaviour	Any treatment that attempts to modulate the sensory intensity component of pain, for example, pharmacological, TNS. SCS, acupuncture, hypnosis distraction/attention control methods
Interference	Failure to complete tasks effectively. Tasks may be incomplete or performed in a degraded manner which is unacceptable to the person	Treatments aimed at restoring functional capacity (physiotherapy and behavioural management)
Identity	The sense of who you are and perhaps more importantly who you might become. Limitations on future achievement of life goals	Treatments that aim to change the individual's relationship to pain and to restore a person's capacity to live according to their life values (e.g. ACT)

TNS = transcutaneous nerve stimulation; SCS = spinal cord stimulation
Adapted from Morley, S (2008).

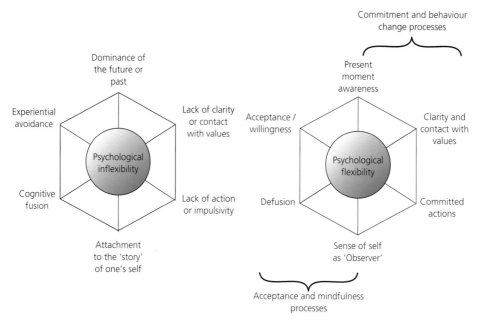

Figure 15.6 The Acceptance and Commitment Therapy Model.

argue that the interruptive effects of pain on daily activity have most impact in terms of psychological functioning according to the degree that the activities are important parts of an individual's identity. An individual who defines himself, for example, as a good father will experience greater impact on mood according to the degree to which his ability to behave 'as a good father would' is disrupted by the pain. If his definition of being a good father involves playing sports with his children and this activity is disrupted by pain, this will have a greater impact than if he, for example, defined himself according to non-disrupted aspects of his life. Individuals who experience more disruption to 'identity-level activities' show greater levels of mood disturbance, even after controlling for pain intensity and activity limitations.

These understandings allow psychological interventions to target those aspects of behaviour and appraisal that are most crucial to identity. We might, for example, help the individual to reappraise what it means to be 'a good father'. 'Good fathering' may be redefined as also including care, support and less active pursuits such as reading stories, feeding and bathing children, and therefore continue to be pursued, even with chronic pain.

Acceptance and Commitment Therapy

Recent developments in psychological therapies have seen a movement away from treatments such as cognitive therapy that emphasise reappraisal and reductions in catastrophising as the target of therapy. Acceptance and Commitment Therapy (ACT) seeks to help individuals to put an end to fruitless attempts to control symptoms such as pain and distressing thoughts and instead to focus on the pursuit of valued life goals, even in the presence of such uncontrollable private experiences (Figure 15.6).

The data for ACT-based interventions in chronic pain are developing rapidly, including one systematic review, with all studies so far reporting significant improvements in distress, disability and

paradoxically pain intensity. ACT-based treatment is particularly well suited to a proportion of chronic pain sufferers who persistently avoid engaging in valued activities in order to keep control over their pain. Whilst appraisal-based models are undoubtedly helpful in understanding and helping chronic pain patients, the introduction of concepts such as acceptance adds an extra dimension to our knowledge of important psychological factors in chronic pain disability and rehabilitation.

Efficacy of psychological therapies for chronic pain

It is now clear from meta-analyses studies of randomised controlled trial data, that behavioural- and cognitive-based therapies are effective in helping people to live more successfully with chronic pain (Table 15.3).

Compared to waiting list controls, moderate effect sizes are seen for cognitive and behavioural treatments in terms of reduced pain, better coping, reduced depression, greater activity and improved social role functioning.

The influence of other healthcare providers

Whilst psychological treatments such as CBT and ACT require specialist training and expertise to deliver, all healthcare providers may apply some of the knowledge of psychological factors to their own work with chronic pain patients. It is clear that patients' beliefs influence their trajectory from acute to chronic pain. Table 15.4 shows a summary of the factors that might lead a healthcare provider to consider whether a patient is at relatively greater risk of developing a chronic pain problem.

Table 15.3 Effect sizes of psychological interventions in chronic pain.

Reference	Population	Trials (n)	Treatment Comparison	Outcome Variable	Effect Size	95% CI	p
Hoffman et al. (2007)	Low back pain	21 (352)	Any psychological therapy versus WLC	Pain intensity	0.52	0.23–0.82	<.001
		21 (288)		Quality of Life	0.39	−0.04–0.82	<.10
		4 (256)	CBT versus WLC	Pain Intensity	0.62	0.25–0.98	<.001
Ostelo et al.(2005)	Low back pain	21 (66*)	Relaxation versus WLC	Pain Intensity	1.16	0.47–1.85	nr
		21 (66*)	CBT versus WLC	Pain Intensity	0.06	0.10–1.09	nr
Dixon et al.(2007)	Chronic Arthritis	27 (3409)	CBT versus control**	Pain Intensity	0.18	0.09–0.26	<0.01
				Anxiety	0.28	0.11–0.46	<0.001
				Depression	0.21	0.05–0.36	<0.01
				Physical Disability	0.15	0.06–0.24	<0.01
				Psychosocial Disability	0.25	0.10–0.40	<0.001
				Active Coping	0.72	00.49–0.94	<0.001
				Self-efficacy	0.18	0.03–0.34	<0.05
Vowles & McCracken (2008)	Mixed pain population	1*** (171)	ACT versus WLC	Pain Intensity	0.70	nr	<0.001
				Depression	1.3	nr	<0.001
				Pain Anxiety	1.0	nr	<0.001
				Physical Disability	0.80	nr	<0.001
				Acceptance	1.8	nr	<0.001
Morley et al. (1999)	Mixed pain population	25 (1672)	CBT or BT versus WLC	Pain Intensity	0.40	0.22–0.58	<0.001
				Depression	0.36	0.13–0.59	<0.001
				Distress	0.52	0.19–0.84	<0.001
				Cognitive Coping	0.51	0.27–0.78	<0.001
				Increased Activity	0.46	0.25–0.72	<0.001
				Social Function	0.60	0.44–0.76	<0.001

*median n of 21 trials (range 17–161); ** control conditions were either Attention Control, TAU, or WLC; ***This is a report of a routine effectiveness trial, rather than an RCT; nr = not reported, ACT = Acceptance and Commitment Therapy

Table 15.4 Psychosocial risk factors for development of chronic pain.

Level A Evidence: (At least two good prospective studies)
- Distress/Anxiety
- Mood Disturbance/Depression
- Passive Coping – resting, relying heavily on others, praying and hoping
- Belief that pain must mean damage
- Avoidance of activities
- Catastrophising – Ruminating, worry, a sense of personal helplessness
- Self-perceived poor physical health

Beliefs about pain influence the patient's journey through the healthcare system, and healthcare providers are in a powerful position potentially to influence those beliefs. The information and advice given by healthcare providers and the way in which it is delivered can be a powerful influence on patient's beliefs. In general, early resumption of normal activities in a graded way and giving patients clear messages about the actual risk of harm to themselves will be useful in countering fear related beliefs and avoidance behaviour.

Summary

Identifying those at risk and offering assertive multidisciplinary treatment is one way of reducing the likelihood of individuals

becoming more disabled, distressed and depressed. Where mood disorders are detected in persons with longstanding or persistent pain, assertive treatment with pharmacotherapy and CBT is indicated. Specialist pain management centres suffer from lack of availability in some countries, although where these are available consideration should be given to this option early in the patient's journey and a full discussion of the concept of self-management and rehabilitation should be had with the patient.

Discussing psychology with a focus on how people respond to persistent pain, rather than psychological factors as 'causing' pain should help both patients and healthcare professionals to engage more meaningfully and potentially more usefully in these kinds of discussions.

References

Crombez, G, Vlaeyen, J, Heuts, PH & Lysens, R (1999) Pain-related fear is more disabling than pain itself: Evidence of the role of pain-related fear in chronic back pain disability. *Pain*, **80**, (1–2), 329–339.

Dixon, KE, Keefe, FJ, Scipio, CD, LisaCaitlin, MP & Abernethy, AP (2007) Psychological interventions for arthritis pain in adults: A meta-analysis. *Health Psychology*, **26** (3), 241–250.

Hoffman, BM, Papas, RK, Chatkoff, DK & Kerns, RD (2007) Meta-analysis for psychological interventions for low back pain. *Health Psychology*, **26** (1), 1–9.

Leventhal, H, Diefenbach, M & Leventhal, EA (1992). Illness cognition: Using common sense to understand treatment adherence and affect cognition interactions. *Cognitive Therapy and Research,* **16** (2), 143–163.

Leeuw, M, Goossens, MEJB, Linton, SJ, Crombez, G, Boersma, K & Vlaeyen, JWS (2007). The Fear-Avoidance Model of musculoskeletal pain: current state of scientific evidence. *Journal of Behavioral Medicine,* **30**, 77–94.

McCracken, L & Eccleston, C (2003) Coping or acceptance: What to do about chronic pain? *Pain,* **105** (1–2), 197–204.

Morley, S (2008) Psychology of pain. *British Journal of Anaesthesia,* **101**, 25–31.

Morley, S, Eccleston, C & Williams, A (1999) Systematic review and meta-analysis of randomized controlled trials of cognitive behaviour therapy and behaviour therapy for chronic pain in adults, excluding headache. *Pain,* **80**, 1–13.

Ostelo RWJG, van Tulder, MW, Vlaeyen, JWS, Linton, SJ, Morley, S & Assendelft, WJJ (2005) Behavioural treatment for chronic low-back pain. *Cochrane Database of Systematic Reviews* **1** (Art. No.: CD002014). doi:10.1002/14651858.

Sullivan, MJL, Bishop, SR & Pivik, J (1995) The pain catastrophizing scale: Development and validation. *Psychological Assessment,* **7** (4), 524–532.

Sullivan, MJ, Thorn, BE, Rodgers, W & Ward, CL (2004) Path model of psychological antecedents to pain experience: Experimental and clinical findings. *Clinical Journal of Pain,* **20** (3), 164–173.

Vlaeyen, JWS & Linton, SJ (2000) Fear-avoidance and its consequences in chronic musculoskeletal pain: A state of the art. *Pain,* **85** (3), 317–332.

Vowles, KE & McCracken, LM (2008) Acceptance and values based action in chronic pain: a study of treatment effectiveness and process. *Journal of Consulting and Clinical Psychology,* **76** (3), 497–407.

Further reading

Dahl, J, Wilson, KG, Luciano, C & Hayes, S (2005) *Acceptance and Commitment Therapy for Chronic Pain.* Reno, NV: Context Press.

Gatchel, RJ & Turk, D (Eds) (2002) *Psychological Approaches to Pain Management: A Practitioner's Handbook,* 2nd edn. New York: Guilford Press.

Stephen Rollnick, S, Miller, WR & Butler, CC (2008). *Motivational Interviewing in Healthcare: Helping Patients Change Behavior.* New York: Guilford Press.

White, C (2001) *Cognitive Behavioural Therapy for Chronic Medical Problems.* Chichester: John Wiley & Sons Ltd.

CHAPTER 16

Interventional Procedures in Pain Management

Dominic Hegarty and Damian Murphy

Department of Anaesthesia and Pain Medicine, Cork University Hospital, Cork, Ireland

---

> **OVERVIEW**
>
> - Interventional procedures in conjunction with a multidisciplinary pain management programme can help improve patient outcome
> - Accurate patient evaluation and selection, taking into consideration the patient's unique presentation of symptoms and overall health status is very import in choosing a suitable intervention
> - Interventional management should start by using the least invasive intervention most likely to provide adequate pain relief before considering more advanced procedures
> - Clear analgesic goals, with regard to clinical outcome, should be discussed with the patient in advance so as to optimise patient satisfaction

Introduction

Chronic non-cancer pain is a common clinical condition afflicting many people, with a significant proportion of them experiencing some form of functional disability (Chapter 1). When pharmacological therapy or conventional surgery fails to control pain adequately or when patients have intolerable side effects to drug treatment, the role of invasive interventional procedures may remain an option for the treatment of chronic pain.

The commonest procedures performed in each anatomical area are listed in Table 16.1. Only some of these procedures are examined in detail and the reader is advised to refer to the 'Further reading' list for more information. While many readers may not be actually performing these interventions, it is important to have an understanding of what is involved if referring patients for assessment and consideration of an intervention.

Patient assessment and selection

Irrespective of what intervention is chosen, proper patient evaluation and selection, taking into consideration the patient's unique presentation of symptoms and overall health status, is

very important. Malignancy, infection and fractures are some of the 'red flags' that must be ruled out prior to the formulation and recommendation of treatment management (Chapter 5). By combining the patients' pain history, clinical examination and appropriate radiological and biochemical investigations, it is possible to choose a suitable intervention for each patient.

General complications

While the benefits of interventional pain strategies are attractive for any symptomatic patient, there are potential risks and complications that should be considered when planning patient management (Figure 16.1). For example, anticoagulation may increase the risks of bleeding, and this should be considered against the potential benefits.

Pharmacological intervention

The most commonly drugs used for interventional procedures include corticosteroids and local anaesthetics (lignocaine and bupivacaine). Steroids relieve pain by reducing inflammation, blocking transmission of nociceptive C-fibre input and inhibiting the action of phospholipase A2, both responsible for cell membrane injury and oedema. Due to the risk of complications associated with prolonged use, corticosteroids for interventional procedures are administered not more than three to four times a year. Local anaesthetics are used to confirm appropriate medication delivery and to provide temporary relief until the corticosteroids reach their therapeutic levels.

Non-pharmacological intervention

Radio frequency or pulsed radio frequency lesioning of nerves or ganglion is a neurodestructive technique that uses continuous heat or radio waves to produce controlled tissue destruction (thermocoagulation). These interventions modulate pain transmission without causing clinical signs of nerve damage. Although pain relief is also temporary because of axon regeneration, multiple controlled trials have shown strong evidence in providing lasting relief for some pain syndromes such as facet joint pain.

ABC of Pain, First edition. Edited by Lesley A Colvin and Marie Fallon.
© 2012 Blackwell Publishing Ltd. Published 2012 by Blackwell Publishing Ltd.

Table 16.1 Common interventional procedures used in each region of the body.

Intervention	Head/Neck region	Thorax Region	Lumbar Region	Pelvic Region
Myofascial blocks	Trigger points of cervical muscles		Trigger points Psoas Major muscle Quadratus Lumborum muscle	
Somatic nerve blocks	Trigeminal Ganglion Maxillary nerve block Mandibular nerve block Glossopharyngeal nerve block Greater & Lesser occipital nerve blocks	Intercostal nerve block Suprascapular nerve block	Lumbar Plexus Block Iliohypogastric nerve Ilioinguinal nerve Genitofemoral nerve	Pudendal Nerve block
Sympathetic block	Sphenopalatine Ganglion block Stellate Ganglion block	T2/T3 Sympathetic block Splanchnic nerve block	Celiac Ganglion block Lumbar Sympathetic block	Hypogastric plexus block Ganglion of Impar block
Spinal injection	Cervical Epidural Cervical Cordotomy Third Occipital nerve block Cervical selective nerve root block	Thoracic Epidural Doral Root entry zone lesioning (DREZ)	Lumbar Epidural Selective Nerve root block Lumbar Discography	Sacral/caudal epidural Sacral Nerve root injection
Joint injection	Temporomandibular Joint Atlanto-occipital Joint Cervical Facets/medial branch block	Thoracic Facets/medial branch block	Lumbar Facet/medial branch block	Sacroiliac joint

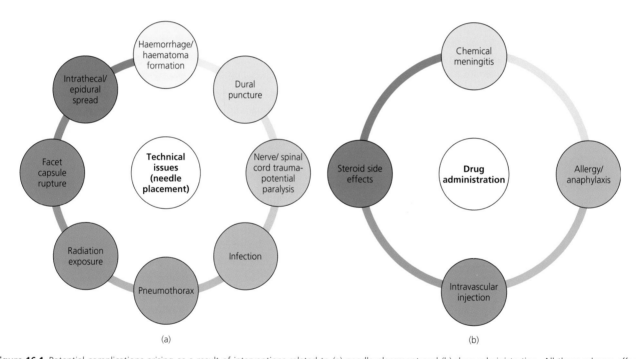

Figure 16.1 Potential complications arising as a result of interventions related to (a) needle placement and (b) drug administration. All these adverse effects, however, are rare and often minor.

Myofascial trigger point injections

Indications

There is no agreement on the definition or valid diagnostic criteria of trigger points in chronic pain. Typically, patients complain of muscle pain and examination often identities a point (a trigger point) that is painful on compression and may produce referred pain, motor dysfunction, and/or autonomic phenomena. Many studies have investigated the efficacy of treating trigger point pain using steroids, dry-needling, Botox and antidepressants with varying results.

Technique

Under sterile conditions the tender point is injected with a combination of either steroid and local anaesthetic, or botulinum toxin. Ultrasound visualisation has been used to help guide the deposition of the agents in the correct muscle layer.

Specific complications

These are relatively straightforward to carry out, but accurate localisation and injection of deep muscle may be problematic and the blind nature of needle advancement increases the risks.

Facet joint injection

Indications

Facet joints have been implicated in 15–45% of patients with back pain and 54–60% of patients with neck pain (but see Chapter 5). Described as dull, stiff or achy pain it is exacerbated by movements that compress the joints (extension, rotation). While pain in the lumbar facet joints radiates typically to the buttocks and upper posterior thigh, and cervical facet joint pain presents with headache, shoulder or mid-back pain, the location of referred pain cannot be used reliably to infer the exact spinal level where the pathology is situated. Unfortunately, facet joint pain cannot be diagnosed consistently by clinical examination or by imaging studies.

Technique

With the patient prone and under fluoroscopic guidance, local anaesthetic (bupivacaine) and corticosteroid are injected around the facet joint (Figures 16.2 and 16.3). A 50% reduction in pain after injection is considered a true positive. A single intra-articular injection results in short-term relief (fewer than six weeks) in 46–75% of patients while long-term relief (six weeks or longer) is seen in 20–36% of the patients. Thus, this intervention is both practical and cost efficient as it is diagnostic as well as therapeutic.

Denervation of the facet joint may be offered to prolong the analgesic effect and this is achieved by pulsed radio frequency of

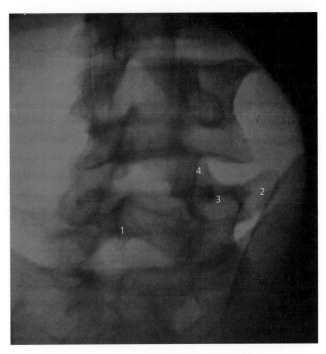

Figure 16.3 Facet joints and medial branch block. The figure shows the oblique radiograph view of the lumbar spine to identify the medial branch (3) and facet joint (4). The 'black dot' at the junction between the transverse process (2) and the facet joint (4) is the target point for a medial branch injection (3). 1 = spinous process.

radio-frequency (RF) thermoablation – a neurodestructive process that involves heating and eventual destruction of nerves supplying the joint (Figure 16.4). However, the duration of pain relief is only extended beyond that from a non-destructive technique and is often not life-long.

Specific complications

Complications of RF neurotomy, although uncommon, can include cutaneous hyperaesthesia or dysaesthesia, neuritis, neurogenic inflammation, anaesthesia dolorosa and deafferentation pain. Excessive burning of tissue outside the target area may also cause escalation of pain.

Epidural steroid injections

Indications

Epidural or selective nerve root blocks using local anaesthetic can be used to confirm the source of radicular pain in 45–100% of cases, especially when imaging studies suggest multiple nerve root involvement. When combined with steroids, such interventions are therapeutic as well, with significant relief lasting for two months or more in 30% of patients with reports of improvement in functional ability in 75% of patients. The majority of studies report strong evidence for short-term improvement and moderate evidence for long-term improvement in managing lumbar and cervical nerve root pain. The data suggest that epidurals have a low incidence of major complications (1.8 per 100 000).

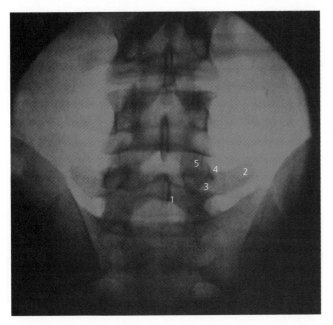

Figure 16.2 Lumbar spine radiograph with labelled landmarks. The figure shows the posterior-anterior radiograph of the lumbar spine with the key landmarks labelled. 1 = spinous process, 2 = transverse process, 3 = pedicle and area of the medial branch, 4 = superior articular process, 5 = inferior articular process of the lumbar vertebrae.

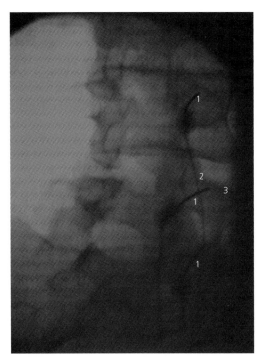

Figure 16.4 Medial branch block and radiofrequency. The figure shows the left oblique radiographic view for the final needles position for L3, L4 and L5 medial branch blocks and radiofrequency. The needles (1) are positioned to lie along the groove formed by the junction of the transverse process (2) and the superior articularis process (3).

Technique

Clinicians may opt to identify the epidural spaced using fluoroscopy and then advance the Touhy needle using a loss of resistance technique (Figure 16.5). Others may choose to use fluoroscopic guidance to advance the Touhy needle slowly and use radio-opaque contrast to confirm the correct placement.

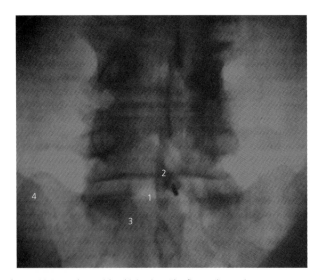

Figure 16.5 Lumbar epidural injection. The figure shows the posterior-anterior radiograph view for the final position of a Touhy epidural needle (black dot) positioned in the L5/S1 interlaminar space (1). 2 = spinous process, 3 = sacrum, 4 = iliac crest.

Specific complications

A dural puncture, with a subsequent post-dural puncture headache, may be higher in those with previous spinal surgery, due to the scarring within the epidural space and adhesion of the dura to the posterior elements. An epidural haematoma or abscess is rare but can lead to significant spinal cord compression.

Selective nerve root injection

Indications

Selective nerve root blocks are used to evaluate and/or treat the cause of pain where clinical symptoms suggest radicular involvement but the precise mechanism may not be clear and MRI may or may not reveal the aetiology. Selective lumbar nerve root injections have a high sensitivity (100%) and specificity 90%.

Technique

The proposed affected nerve root is identified using fluoroscopy. A combination of local anaesthetic and steroids is used to diagnosis and treat the pain (Figures 16.6 and 16.7).

Specific complications

Inadvertent nerve contact can lead to mechanical nerve root damage. Intrathecal injection, facial flushing, leg pain and intraoperative hypertension have been reported infrequently.

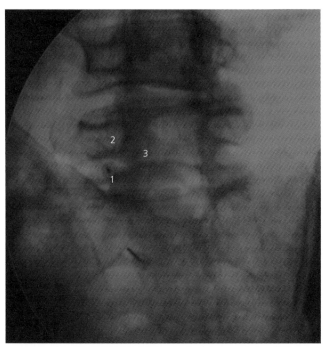

Figure 16.6 Selective nerve root block. The figure shows the right oblique radiograph of the lumbar spine with the needle in the final position for a selective nerve root block. The needle tip (1) lies directly inferior to the pedicle (2) and inferolateral to the pars intericularis (3). The needle is advanced to meet the vertebral body and the position checked with a lateral radiograph before injection of steroid.

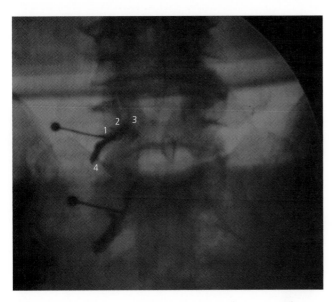

Figure 16.7 Selective nerve root block with radiographic contrast. The figure shows the posterior-anterior radiograph view of the lumbar spine following selective nerve root injection (after radiographic contrast). The needle tip (1) is in the final position and lies directly inferior to the pedicle (2) and the contrast extends to the lateral epidural space beneath the pedicle (towards 3). The contrast also extends along the lateral aspect of the nerve roots as it exits the intervertebral foramen (towards 4)

Lumbar sympathetic block

Indications

Lumbar sympathetic block is effective in 48–80% of patients with certain chronic pain syndromes involving the lower extremities. Some of these conditions include complex regional pain syndrome, ischaemic pain and painful diabetic neuropathy.

Technique

With the patient prone a needle is advanced towards the anterior border of the L3 vertebral body under fluoroscopic guidance. Radio-opaque contrast confirms the correct needle position before 10 ml of bupivacaine and steroid is injected.

Specific complications

Intravascular injection and resultant toxic levels of local anaesthetic can occur.

Genitofemoral neuralgia is reported in 5–20% of patients. Other complications include transient post-sympathectomy neuropathic pain in the anterolateral proximal lower limb, damage to the kidney and ureter, and ejaculatory failure. These complications are seen more commonly after neurolytic blockade.

Intrathecal drug delivery

Indications

Intrathecal drug delivery is an alternative way to manage pain associated with cancer, multiple sclerosis and other non-malignant pain, such as failed back syndrome, complex regional pain syndromes, phantom limb pain and painful spasticity. It provides the options of using drugs at high concentrations without the limitations imposed by the intolerable side effects associated with oral, transdermal, subcutaneous or intravenous routes.

Drugs used for intrathecal delivery include opioids, clonidine, baclofen and local anaesthetics. Evidence for implantable intrathecal drug delivery systems is strong for short-term improvement in neuropathic pain and moderate for long-term management of chronic pain. It can be extremely effective in the management of complex cancer pain, with some evidence that it may even improve survival.

Technique

Usually, the intrathecal system is placed under general anaesthesia, or local anaesthesia with sedation, with full surgical precautions. Fluoroscopy can be used to confirm/identify the epidural space, after which the intrathecal catheter is advanced. The catheter is tunnelled subcutaneously and connected to a continuous analgesic delivery pump, which is sited in a subcutaneous pocket usually created in the hypochondrium or iliac fossa (Figure 16.8). Continuing review with pump refills at appropriate intervals is always required.

Complications

Complications can either be device- or drug-related or both. Device-related complications include wound infection or catheter breakage/migration. Drug-related complications include dosing/programming errors, pump filling errors and the spectrum of opioid-related side effects, including nausea, sedation, urinary retention, pruritus and respiratory depression. These side effects are minimised through patient monitoring and careful dose adjustments, and double checking the settings before the patient's departure from the clinic. In general, in a stable patient who begins to have side effects shortly after the pump refill, the programming should be double-checked promptly. A rare complication is granuloma formation at the catheter tip.

Spinal cord stimulation (neuromodulation)

Indications

A spinal cord stimulator (SCS) is used to deliver mild electrical pulses directly to the spinal cord or nerve fibres. It is indicated when other pain management options have been exhausted. Painful conditions that may respond to SCS include chronic angina, failed back surgery syndrome, complex regional pain syndrome, severe ischaemic limb pain secondary to peripheral vascular disease, and peripheral neuropathic pain. Evidence for SCS in failed back surgery syndrome and complex regional pain syndrome is strong for short-term relief (less than one year) and moderate for long-term relief (more than one year).

Technique

SCS involves the placement of electrodes in the epidural space aiming to place them on/next to the surface of the dura mater

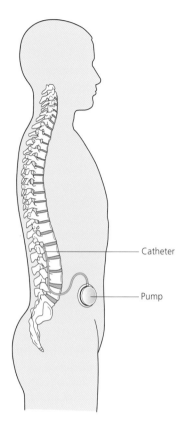

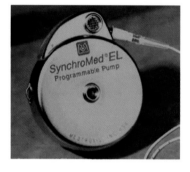

Catheter

Pump

Figure 16.8 Intrathecal drug delivery system. The figure illustrates the insertion set up of an intrathecal drug delivery system pump. The catheter is inserted into the epidural space either under direct vision or with radiological guidance. The catheter is then tunnelled subcutaneously and connected to a continuous analgesic delivery pump, which is sited in a subcutaneous pocket created in the hypochondrium or iliac fossa.

overlying the target level of the cord. Electrodes may be inserted either percutaneously, with the patient able to localise correct placement by identifying appropriate parasthesia, or using an open technique (more commonly performed by neurosurgeons) under general anaesthesia. Under fluoroscopic guidance and with on-table stimulation further manoeuvring of the electrodes can be made to ensure appropriate paraesthesia coverage. The leads are tunnelled subcutaneously and connected to an electronic impulse generator. This device is placed in a subcutaneous pocket created in the hypochondrium or iliac fossa. Post-operative antibiotics may be prescribed (Figure 16.9).

Specific complications

Complications with SCS range from infection, haematoma, seroma, nerve damage, lack of appropriate paraesthesia coverage, post-dural puncture headache, electrode migration or failure, paralysis and nerve injury.

Unfortunately, in order to confirm correct electrode placement general anaesthesia can only be provided once this part of the procedure is complete and this can be difficult for some patients. Acute nociceptive pain immediately following the procedure can be expected and analgesia should be prescribed as appropriate.

Summary

It must be recognised that a multidisciplinary approach to chronic pain is very important to maximise patient outcome. Interventional

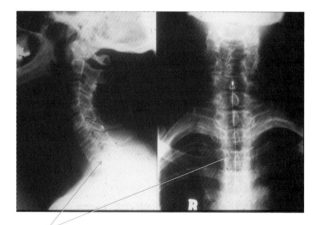

Electrode: situated in the epidural space, in the midline to avoid nerve root irritation

Figure 16.9 Radiographic appearance of dorsal column stimulator electrode used for chronic end stage angina.

procedures can have a valuable role to play in the overall management of chronic pain. However, correctly choosing a suitable intervention is critical to ensure the overall benefit for each patient because each procedure is not without its own complications.

Further Reading

Boswell, MV, Trescot, AM, Datta, S, Schultz, DM, Hansen, HC, Abdi, S, *et al.* (2007) Interventional techniques: evidence-based practice guidelines in the management of chronic spinal pain. *Pain Physician*, **10**, 7–111.

Cook, TM, Counsell, D & Wildsmith, AW (2009) Major complications of central neuraxial block: report on the Third National Audit Project of the Royal College of Anaesthetists. *British Journal of Anaesthesia*, **102** (2), 179–190.

Nocom, G, Ho, KY & Perumal, M (2009) Interventional Management of Chronic Pain. *Ann Acad Med Singapore*, **38**, 150–155.

Raj, PP, Lou, L, Erdine, S, *et al.* (2008) *Interventional Pain Management: image guided procedures*, 2nd edn. Philadelphia, PA: Saunders-Elsvier.

Turner, JA, Loeser, JD, Deyo, RA & Sanders, SB (2004) Spinal cord stimulation for patients with failed back surgery syndrome or complex regional pain syndrome: A systemic review of effectiveness and complications. *Pain*, **108**, 137–147.

CHAPTER 17

The Role of Physiotherapy in Pain Management

Paul J Watson

Department of Health Sciences, University of Leicester, Leicester, UK

OVERVIEW

- Physiotherapy is delivered as a package of care involving different elements
- There is good evidence for the effectiveness of manual therapy, exercise and educational/behavioural modification approaches in the management of subacute and chronic musculoskeletal pain
- Combining manual therapy and exercise may be more effective that one element alone
- The evidence for TENS is conflicting but it may provide a medication sparing function in some conditions
- Physiotherapy aims to maximise a patient's participation in activities of daily living, social functioning and work

Introduction

The symptom of pain is one of the commonest reasons for consulting a physiotherapist and the treatment of pain, especially musculoskeletal pain, occupies the majority of clinician time in a busy outpatient department. A physiotherapist can be involved at all durations of injury, from acute injury on the sports field to chronic pain management programmes.

Physiotherapy covers a variety of treatments, some which are well supported by evidence and others which have not been subjected to close scrutiny. It would be a mistake to see physiotherapy as consisting of one or other of these treatments, rather than a package of care (Figure 17.1). At its best physiotherapy is a package of rehabilitation but time constraints and the knowledge, beliefs and experience of the individual therapist can mitigate against the provision of optimal treatment. Most physiotherapy is concerned with the subacute and, especially, the chronic phase of injury; the techniques and treatment are discussed further here.

Physiotherapy in acute injury

The aim of physiotherapy for acute pain is to manage the underlying inflammatory process to encourage healing and early restoration of function.

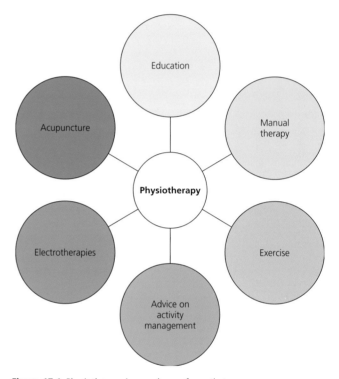

Figure 17.1 Physiotherapy is a *package of care* that may encompass a range of therapies, with some examples shown here.

Movement restriction is recommended in the very early stage of an acute injury and this is achieved by the use of splints and non-elastic strapping or bandaging (Figures 17.2 and 17.3). The latter also provides compression to help reduce swelling but must be applied carefully and reviewed regularly to prevent further complications. Cold therapy is applied immediately to reduce pain and swelling. At its simplest cold therapy is ice alone but there are a number of sophisticated cold therapy devices which can be incorporated into splints to provide both cold therapy and compression.

Ice may be applied repeatedly over one or two weeks to keep swelling under control. It is often applied after exercise in the early stages of rehabilitation. Ice cools the tissue and lowers tissue metabolism in the immediate stages after injury, it reduces hypoxic cell death and relieves pain through reducing neuronal activity. Ice must be applied early; a delay of 24 hours will reduce the

ABC of Pain, First edition. Edited by Lesley A Colvin and Marie Fallon.
© 2012 Blackwell Publishing Ltd. Published 2012 by Blackwell Publishing Ltd.

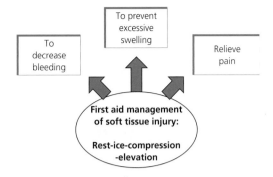

Figure 17.2 First aid in the management of acute soft tissue pain.

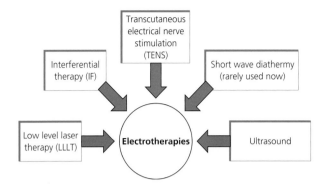

Figure 17.4 Electrotherapies used in the treatment of pain.

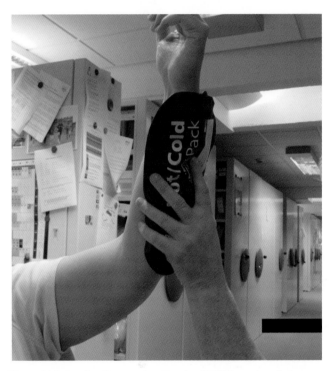

Figure 17.3 Rest, Ice, Compression, Elevation (RICE) for acute soft tissue injury.

effectiveness of ice therapy. Early mobilisation is recommended once the acute stage of healing starts to subside. This will of course depend on the severity of the injury.

Electrotherapies

A range of electrotherapies can be used in the management of both acute and chronic injury (Figure 17.4). The research evidence for many of these treatments is scant, often with conflicting results. The main problem with the research is the lack of scientific rigour in many of the studies.

Low level laser therapy (LLLT)

Reviews of the literature have suggested that there is some evidence for the use of LLLT in people with chronic joint problems, such as osteoarthritis, and some myofascial pain problems (Figure 17.5).

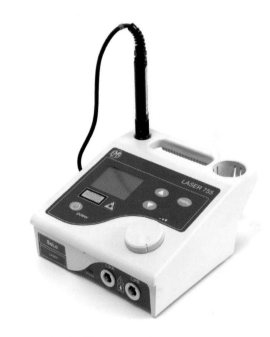

Figure 17.5 A low level laser therapy device.

The mode of action is unclear but laboratory studies have suggested that LLLT can modulate pain through reducing pro-inflammatory cytokines and reduce the development of oedema. The effect on non-specific low back pain and other musculoskeletal pain problems is inconclusive and generally laser therapy has gradually diminished in use, at least in the National Health Service in the United Kingdom, because of a lack of clear evidence of effect.

Transcutaneous Electrical Nerve Stimulation (TENS)

Transcutaneous Electrical Nerve Stimulation (TENS) will be familiar to most clinicians; these small portable devices are easily available and widely used by patients who often buy them from pharmacists. The device emits an electrical current which can be varied. Clinically TENS is considered worth trying in a wide variety of musculoskeletal pain conditions because it is simple to use, has low risk and only a short trial is required to evaluate the effectiveness in an individual patient.

In the acute pain setting, studies have demonstrated no advantage of TENS over routine analgesia in post-operative pain; however, subsequent reviews considering the quality of the clinical application of TENS have concluded there is a medication sparing role for TENS and it could be considered as an adjunct to routine analgesia where patients wish to restrict their medication consumption.

The mechanism of action and practical use of TENS in chronic pain is covered further in Chapter 18.

Interferential therapy

Interferential Therapy (IF) stimulators generate two out of phase currents via two pairs of electrodes, one with a frequency of 1–400 Hz and the other between 2 and 4 KHz (Figure 17.6). It is suggested that these currents interfere with each other to produce a 'beat' frequency which can be delivered to deep tissues. It is proposed that the mechanism of effect is similar to TENS, and indeed in experimental laboratory studies the two are comparable. Most commentators now believe the effect of IF is as a result of the high frequency current. The clinical effectiveness of IF is similar to TENS. The disadvantage of IF is that it is often delivered in an outpatient setting, although devices the patient can wear are available. The common consent is that IF has no advantage over TENS.

Ultrasound

Clinically, therapeutic ultrasound is a high frequency mechanical vibration typically between 0.75 and 3 MHz (Figure 17.7). The action of therapeutic ultrasound is purported to be through an ability to affect the inflammatory process. It is suggested that it promotes the proliferation of fibroblasts and endothelial cells into the damaged area and stimulates myofibroblasts to initiate wound healing. In addition, it may increase protein synthesis and accelerates collagen production, the net result of which is accelerated

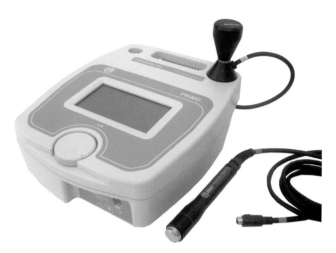

Figure 17.7 A therapeutic ultrasound device.

wound healing. Experimental studies have not demonstrated this to be the case and clinical studies and systematic reviews have not supported a role in increased healing or clinical improvement. As a result the use of ultrasound in acute soft tissue injuries has declined and it is rarely recommended.

Manual therapies

Mobilisation and manipulation of joints and massage of soft tissues are commonly performed for painful conditions. Manipulations (also known as spinal adjustments when applied to the spine) are small amplitude, high velocity thrust manoeuvres near or at the limit of normal movement, and normally cannot be controlled by the patient. Mobilisation in manual therapy involves procedures where the therapist uses hand and fingers to handle tissues to increase the range of motion beyond the passive range of motion or exercise. Mobilisations are low velocity, repetitive and performed in a way that the patient can prevent it being performed.

Joint mobilisation increases range of motion through repeated stretching and deformation of the tissues which increases the extensibility of joint structures. Short-term increased range of motion immediately following manual therapy is well documented. This is probably achieved through alterations in the biomechanical integrity of the tissue and joint structures. Pain relief after both procedures is well documented and is reported in systematic reviews (Box 17.1).

> **Box 17.1 Manipulation to improve joint mobility**
>
> The reasons why joint mobility improves following these procedures include:
>
> - breaking of adhesions between adherent tissues
> - alterations in the extensibility of soft tissue, restoration of normal joint biomechanics
> - repositioning of disrupted intra-articular or intradiscal material
> - altered sympathetic nervous system activity

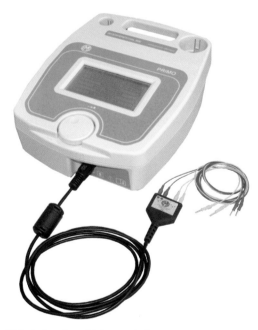

Figure 17.6 An interferential therapy device.

Most of these have been demonstrated in experimental studies although the relationship between these and changes in pain and disability are less clear. Many studies have established that manual therapy is better than placebo and usually better than treatment as usual by a general practitioner in the management of spinal pain and associated disability in the subacute and chronic stages. There is little evidence that regular spinal adjustment prevents the development of pain in pain-free individuals or reduces the frequency of exacerbations in those with recurrent problems.

Exercise therapy

Exercise is one of the basic cornerstones of physiotherapy in painful conditions. Pain frequently restricts movement. In the acute stage this can be desirable; immobilisation to aid repair is frequent in acute pain, especially trauma. Immobilisation for any period reduces the strength and function of muscles, tendon and ligaments. Over time it also leads to impaired neuromuscular coordination, which can lead to biomechanical dysfunction and recurrent injury. Movement restriction is a reduction in physical activity of either the painful area or of the body in general. This may be imposed by the patient due to pain, the belief that movement may cause further pain or injury and often by the advice from others, including healthcare professionals. Restricted physical activity may result in reduced cardiovascular fitness. The degree to which this occurs depends on the patient's physical activity levels before the pain commenced. Those who were not physically active before the onset of their pain may not have any appreciable reduction in activity levels or fitness.

Physical exercise produces stress on the tissues to stimulate tissue remodelling and promote healing if applied appropriately. What kind of exercise to prescribe will depend upon the patient's individual problems (Figure 17.8). A clinical assessment may be relatively straight forward in the case of an acute injury or a very specific diagnosis. The injured tissue can be identified allowing a

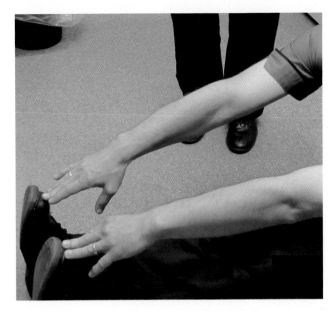

Figure 17.9 Specific stretches can be tailored for individual patients to improve mobility.

specific management strategy focused throughout the healing and rehabilitation process. In the case of pain conditions without a clear cause, such as characterises many musculoskeletal pain conditions, and in the case of chronic pain, especially low back pain, the picture is less clear.

Over the years there have been many specific exercise programmes for common conditions, such as low back and neck pain, but the evidence now demonstrates that general exercise programmes are equally effective in reducing pain and disability in the short term and at long term follow up. General exercise regimes include stretching, strengthening and cardiovascular conditioning exercises. Supervised exercises tailored to the needs of individual patients (with respect to their activity tolerance, previous fitness, required fitness daily activities including work, and any identifiable specific problems) with an emphasis on performing exercises at home appear to be the most effective (Figure 17.9). Short, non-intense exercise programmes appear to be less effective than longer, more intense programmes, at least in the treatment of chronic spinal pain conditions. Providing manual therapy in addition to exercise has been shown to increase the effect of treatment and may even be more cost effective in low back pain.

All exercise programmes should emphasise the need to return to normal physical activities as part of the rehabilitation process.

Behaviour modification

It is well documented that many of the obstacles to rehabilitation and the factors which are predictive of poor outcome following the onset of a painful condition are psychosocial (Figure 17.10).

Physiotherapy interventions, especially when encouraging patients to exercise and return to usual activities, require a considerable trust in the therapist that the activity will not cause harm and that the effort and investment will have a worthwhile outcome.

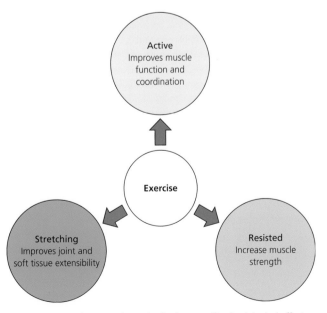

Figure 17.8 Specific types of exercise lead to specific physiological effects.

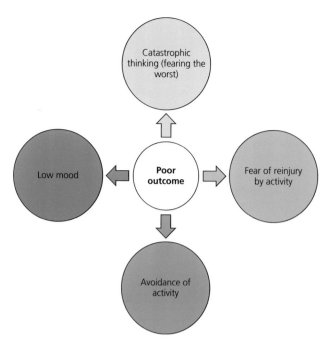

Figure 17.10 Some of the factors that may contribute to a poor outcome in patients with chronic pain.

Patient adherence to advice and rehabilitation programmes can be improved if the patient has a better understanding of their condition, is not afraid that they will cause harm, and can identify success through regaining valued activities.

Most guidelines on the management of painful conditions advocate educating the patient on their condition. Physiotherapists have taken a more systematic approach to this in recent years, emphasising information that is likely to explain pain in terms which are understandable to the patient and which promote a benign view of pain especially chronic pain. In chronic pain conditions where there is no obvious single cause of the pain this can be difficult. Recent studies have demonstrated the importance of education in reducing the fear of reinjury and enhancing participation in activity or previously feared activity through promoting a cognitive shift in the patient's beliefs about their condition. Educational interventions designed to elicit and challenge distorted beliefs about pain, physical activity and, in particular, activities of daily living should be core components of physiotherapy in chronic pain conditions. Reducing fear of activity can reduce disability and increase objective physical performance tasks in people with chronic pain. Sometimes simple educational approaches are insufficient and patients are encouraged to engage systematically in previously feared activities as mini behavioural experiments to reduce specific fears about physical activity.

Avoidance of important activities, including work, and a reduced participation or avoidance of valued activities can increase the risk of developing depression. For this reason, physiotherapy rehabilitation should emphasise returning to these activities as part of the management plan. Patients are encouraged to identify valued activities and set goals to re-engaging in them. There is increasing evidence that physiotherapy interventions which incorporate some simple elements of cognitive behavioural therapy are more effective than routine physiotherapy but the role of these interventions in those deemed at highest risk of poor outcome (based on psychosocial factors) remains to be seen. A limited number of studies have demonstrated that this 'high risk' group only benefits from more intensive, multidisciplinary pain management programmes.

Conclusion

Physiotherapy for pain represents a wide variety of techniques and skills which are rarely delivered in isolation. In recent years there has been a shift from applying hands-on or intervention-based approaches to the identification of risk factors for poor outcome and integrating the management of these, mainly psychosocial factors, into physiotherapy treatment and rehabilitation. Although a reduction in pain remains a key outcome following physiotherapy, a reduction of disability and re-engagement in physical, social and work activities has gained importance.

It is only possible to give the broadest outline of the role of physiotherapy and the reader is directed to the further reading list for more detailed information.

Further reading

Main, CJ, Sullivan, MJL, Watson PJ (2008) *Pain Management: Practical applications of the biopsychosocial perspective in clinical and occupational settings.* Edinburgh: Churchill Livingstone.

Sluka, KA (ed.) (2009) *Pain Mechanisms and Management for the Physical Therapists.* Seattle, WA: IASP Press.

Watson, PJ, Main, CJ & Smeets, RJEM (2010) The Basics: Management and Treatment of Low back pain. In: Mogil, JS (ed.) *Pain 2010 – An Updated Review: Refresher Course Syllabus.* Seattle, WA: IASP Press.

Watson, T (ed.) (2008) *Electrotherapy: evidence-based practice.* Edinburgh: Churchill Livingstone.

CHAPTER 18

The Role of Transcutaneous Electrical Nerve Stimulation (TENS) in Pain Management

Mark I Johnson

Faculty of Health and Social Sciences, Leeds Metropolitan University and Leeds Pallium Research Group, Leeds, UK

OVERVIEW

- Transcutaneous electrical nerve stimulation (TENS) is an inexpensive, self-administered technique with no known potential for overdose

- Clinical research suggests that TENS is useful as an adjunct to pharmacotherapy for acute pain and as a stand-alone treatment for chronic pain

- Pain relief with TENS is maximal when strong non-painful TENS paraesthesiae are experienced beneath the electrodes, so patients may need to administer TENS throughout the day

- TENS selectively activates non-noxious afferents (A-beta) which has been shown to inhibit nociceptor cell activity in the central nervous system

- Acupuncture-like TENS is a form of hyperstimulation which is used for patients who do not respond to conventional TENS

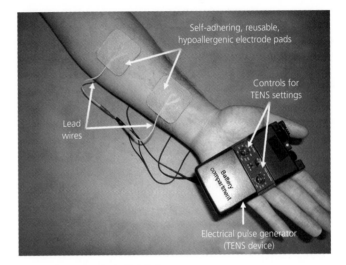

Figure 18.1 A standard TENS device.

Introduction

Transcutaneous electrical nerve stimulation (TENS) is a non-invasive analgesic technique that administers pulsed electrical currents across the intact surface of the skin to activate underlying nerves. A battery powered portable device is used to generate currents and self-adhering conducting pad electrodes are used to deliver the currents through the skin (Figure 18.1). TENS is used as a stand-alone treatment for mild to moderate pain and in combination with drug medication for moderate to severe pain. There is no known potential for overdose and there are few side effects or drug interactions, so patients can self-administer TENS and titrate dosage as required. Effects are generally rapid in onset and offset so patients are encouraged to administer TENS throughout the day. TENS devices are inexpensive and can be purchased without medical prescription in the United Kingdom.

Electric catfish (Malapterurus electricus) and electric rays (Torpedo marmorata) which can generate 300-volt shocks were used by the ancient Egyptians (2500 BC), Greeks (400 BC) and Romans (AD 46) to treat pain (Figure 18.2). The invention of electrostatic machines catalysed the use of electrotherapeutic devices in mainstream medicine in the 19th century.

In 1965, Melzack and Wall suggested that activity in large diameter myelinated afferents (A-beta) could inhibit onward transmission of noxious information in the central nervous system resulting in pain relief akin to 'rubbing pain better'. Percutaneous electrical stimulation of peripheral nerves was shown to reduce chronic neuropathic pain and dorsal column stimulation, a forerunner of spinal cord stimulation, shown to relieve chronic pain. TENS was used to predict the success of spinal cord stimulation implants until it was realised that TENS was a successful modality on its own. Nowadays, a variety of 'TENS-like devices' are available on the market (Johnson, 2001), although the term TENS is generally used to describe stimulation using a 'standard TENS device' (Figure 18.3).

Techniques and mechanism of action

Users select different TENS settings and electrode positions in order to activate different types of peripheral nerve fibre (Box 18.1).

ABC of Pain, First edition. Edited by Lesley A Colvin and Marie Fallon.
© 2012 Blackwell Publishing Ltd. Published 2012 by Blackwell Publishing Ltd.

Box 18.1 **TENS techniques**

TENS technique	Physiological intention	Settings	Electrode location	Regimen
Conventional TENS (Low intensity, high frequency)	Selective stimulation of low threshold afferents (A-beta)	High frequency (>50pps) Low intensity (non-painful paraesthesiae) Short pulse duration (50–200µs)	At the painful region or main nerve bundle arising from painful region	Whenever in pain
Acupuncture-like TENS (High intensity, low frequency)	Stimulation of high threshold cutaneous and muscle afferents (A-delta)	Low frequency (<5pps or five bursts per second) High intensity (just below pain threshold or above motor threshold) Long pulse duration (100–400µs)	Trigger points, acupuncture points, or at the painful region	~30minutes at a time
Intense TENS (High intensity, high frequency)	Stimulation of high threshold cutaneous afferents (A-delta)	High frequency (>50pps) High intensity (above pain threshold) Long pulse duration (100–400µs)	At the painful region	~15minutes at a time

Conventional TENS

The physiological intention of TENS, in its conventional form, is to selectively stimulate A-beta afferents in pain-related dermatomes (Figure 18.4). Extracellular recordings from spinal cord neurones in anaesthetised rats and cats have shown that TENS delivered to somatic receptive fields inhibits noxious evoked responses in sensitised wide dynamic range cells immediately and one hour after stimulation. This inhibition remains after spinal cord transection, suggesting segmental neural circuitry. TENS reduces aspartate and glutamate levels in the spinal cord via the release of the inhibitory neurotransmitter gamma-aminobutyric acid (GABA).

Large diameter afferents have lower thresholds of excitation than their small diameter counterparts, so A-beta afferents are selectively activated by titrating TENS pulse amplitude. A strong, comfortable, non-painful paraesthesia beneath the electrodes is indicative of A-beta activation and is achieved using low intensity currents. Large diameter afferents have short refractory periods and high rates of impulse generation. Hence, high frequency TENS may produce a stronger afferent barrage and stronger segmental inhibition. Low frequency TENS has been shown to involve mu opioid receptors and high frequency TENS delta opioid receptors in animal studies. Claims about optimal pulse frequencies, durations and patterns in humans are based on poor quality research, so patients are encouraged to adjust settings to find the most comfortable settings for their pain at that moment in time.

Acupuncture-like TENS (AL-TENS)

AL-TENS is a form of hyperstimulation first described Sjölund and colleagues. The physiological intention of AL-TENS is to activate high threshold cutaneous and muscle afferents (A-delta) which prolongs segmental nociceptor cell inhibition by up to 2 hours. AL-TENS has been shown to activate nuclei in the midbrain periaqueductal grey and rostral ventromedial medulla associated with descending pain inhibitory pathways which synapse at all levels of the spinal cord. This leads to extrasegmental analgesia (Figure 18.5). AL-TENS increases central levels of opioids, serotonin and noradrenaline, which have a key role in inhibiting onward transmission of noxious information in the spinal cord.

AL-TENS is administered using high intensity, low frequency currents. AL-TENS is often delivered to generate non-painful muscle twitches because A-delta muscle afferent activity has been shown to generate larger inhibition than cutaneous afferents. The user titrates TENS pulse amplitude to the desired intensity; low frequency trains or bursts (2–4 Hz) of high frequency pulses (100–200 pps) are often used, as they are more comfortable than single pulses delivered at low frequency. Electrodes are positioned in pain-related dermatomes, myotomes, acupuncture points and trigger points. Patients administer AL-TENS less frequently than conventional TENS, for example 20 minutes, three times a day.

Intense TENS

Intense TENS is a form of counter-irritation and activates diffuse noxious inhibitory controls. The physiological intention of intense TENS is to activate high threshold cutaneous afferents (A-delta) at intensities above pain threshold. High frequency pulses (up to 200 pps) and longer pulse durations that activate small diameter fibres at lower pulse amplitudes are used. Electrodes are positioned in pain-related dermatomes. Intense TENS is delivered for short periods of time for minor procedures such as wound dressing and suture removal.

Mechanism of action

TENS antidromically activates peripheral nerves and TENS-induced impulses have been shown to extinguish afferent impulses arising from peripheral structures via a 'busy line-effect'. TENS-induced A-beta activity will block large diameter afferent input that may be contributing to pain and TENS-induced A-delta activity will block small diameter afferent input from nociceptors (Figure 18.6).

Practicalities

Patients should undergo a pain assessment before receiving TENS for the first time. Conventional TENS is selected in the first instance

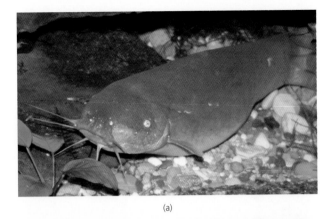

(a)

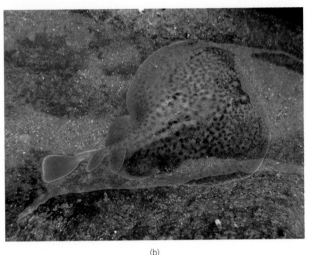

(b)

Figure 18.2 Natural sources of electrical pain modulation. a) Malapterurus electricus – Electric Catfish. b) Torpedo marmorata – Marbled Electric Ray. Photos courtesy of Stan Shebs.

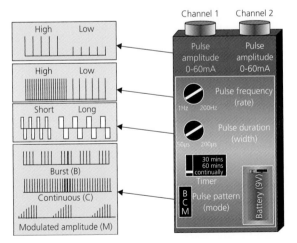

Figure 18.3 Output characteristics of a standard TENS device. Differences in design between manufacturers are often minor and cosmetic.

for most patients and AL-TENS used when patients do not respond to conventional TENS. A supervised trial of conventional TENS is necessary to ensure the patient receives clear, simple instructions on TENS and that they are sufficiently competent in TENS use (Box 18.2).

Box 18.2 **A simple protocol for conventional TENS**

1 Check contraindications and test skin for normal sensation
2 Initial TENS settings adjusted when device is switched off

- Pulse pattern (mode) = continuous
- Pulse frequency (rate) = mid-range (80–100pps)
- Pulse duration (width) = mid-range (100–200μs)
- Timer (if available) = continuous

3 Position electrodes at site of pain or over main nerve bundle
4 Connect electrode lead wires to TENS device and switch on
5 Slowly increase intensity until patient reports first TENS 'tingling' sensation
6 Slowly increase intensity until patient reports a strong but comfortable tingling sensation
7 Experiment with settings while maintaining the strong but comfortable tingling
8 Adjust duration of stimulation according to need

During conventional TENS maximal pain relief occurs when a strong but comfortable electrical paraesthesia is perceived beneath the electrodes, so patients may need to leave TENS 'switched on' throughout the day to obtain continuing pain relief. The user titrates TENS pulse amplitude to the desired intensity and needs to adjust amplitude regularly to maintain the strong comfortable intensity. Painful TENS paraesthesiae are not the desired outcome for conventional TENS.

Electrodes should be positioned on healthy sensate skin; this should be checked prior to application. In general, electrodes are positioned on relevant dermatomes and paraesthesia directed into the painful area (Figure 18.7). However, this is not appropriate in the presence of mechanical allodynia because TENS may exacerbate the pain. Alternative positions can be used, such as along the main nerves proximal to the site of pain, paravertebrally at appropriate segments or at contralateral 'mirror' sites.

Over half of patients may respond to TENS and many of these continue to become long-term successful users. However, the effects of repeated daily use of TENS may decline over time. This may be because of a worsening pain problem, nervous system habituation and/or the development of opioid tolerance. Changing TENS settings, electrode placements and treatment schedules, or even withdrawing TENS temporarily, may resolve the problem. TENS can be used whilst going to sleep provided the device has a timer so that it switches off automatically. Dual channel TENS devices with four electrodes are used for large or multiple pains.

Contraindications, precautions and adverse events

Manufacturers list cardiac pacemakers, pregnancy and epilepsy as contraindications because it may be difficult to exclude TENS as a potential cause of a problem from a legal perspective. However, the UK Chartered Society of Physiotherapy guidelines for the use of electrophysical agents list cardiac pacemakers and bleeding disorders as a contraindication and pregnancy and epilepsy as a

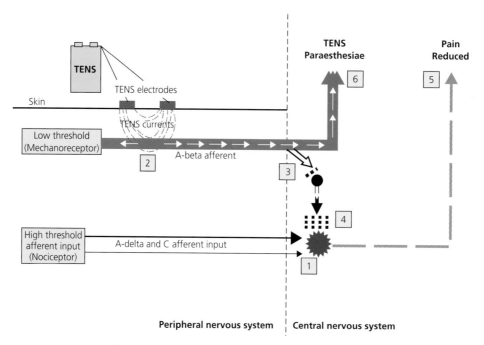

Figure 18.4 Segmental action of conventional TENS. White arrows indicate TENS-induced impulses leading to segmental analgesia. Nociceptive afferent input causes activity in second order nociceptive transmission cells in the central nervous system [1] which leads to pain. Activation of large diameter non-noxious afferents by TENS [2] activates interneurones [3] which release inhibitory neurotransmitters such as GABA and reduce activity in second order nociceptive transmission cells [4]. Nociceptive input to the brain declines resulting in pain relief [5]. TENS-induced activity in non-noxious transmitting pathways results in a sensation of electrical paraesthesiae [6].

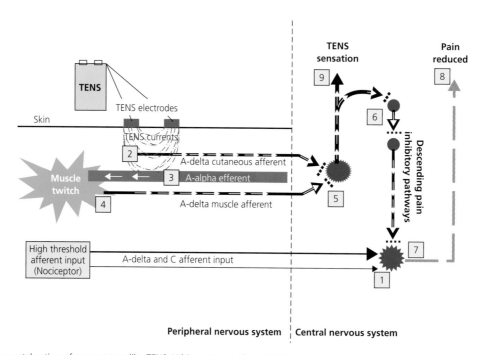

Figure 18.5 Extrasegmental action of acupuncture-like TENS. White arrows indicate TENS-induced impulses leading to extrasegmental analgesia. Nociceptive afferent input causes activity in second order nociceptive transmission cells [1] which leads to pain. Higher intensity TENS activates A-delta afferents directly [2] and/or motor neurones leading to a muscle twitch [3]. Small diameter muscle afferent activity from the muscle twitch [4] activates central ascending pathways [5], which excite descending pain inhibitory pathways [6] and inhibition of second order nociceptive transmission cells [7]. Nociceptive input to the brain declines resulting in pain relief [8]. TENS induced activity results in sensations of electrical 'twitching' [9].

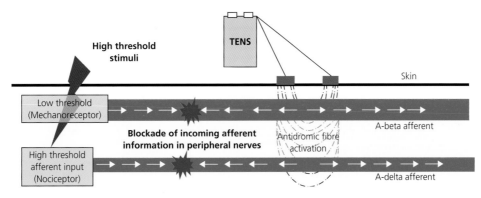

Figure 18.6 Peripheral action of TENS. White arrows indicate TENS-induced impulses leading to peripheral blockade. Grey arrows indicate afferent impulses arising from peripheral structures.

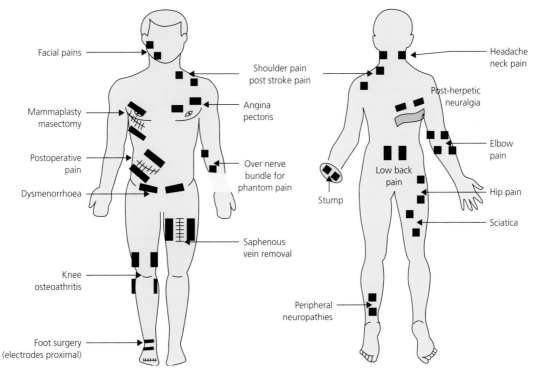

Figure 18.7 TENS electrode positions.

Box 18.3 **Precautions when using TENS**

CI – Contraindicated	Comment
Cardiac Pacemakers (CI)	Check with patient's cardiologist.
Cardiovascular conditions	Liaise with cardiologist, apply with caution and monitor progress frequently. Can be used for angina.
Pregnancy (Local CI)	Check with patient's obstetrician and midwife. Can be used during childbirth.
Epilepsy (Local CI)	Check with from patient's neurologist.
Malignancy (Local CI)	Check with patient's oncologist or palliative care specialist.
Allodynia/Hyperalgesia (Local CI)	TENS may, but not always, exacerbate the pain. Apply TENS on skin with normal sensation in first instance.
Non-adherent patients	Assess patient for competency

local contraindication, that is electrodes should not be positioned over abdomen or head, respectively. Electrodes should not be positioned over an active tumour for a patient whose tumour is treatable. Risk–benefit decisions are at the discretion of the medical practitioner (Box 18.3).

Serious adverse events from TENS appear to be rare. Some patients experience mild autonomic responses and minor skin irritation beneath electrodes. TENS can interfere with monitoring equipment and should not be placed close to transdermal drug delivery systems. Children as young as four years of age can tolerate TENS provided they are able to comprehend instructions. A point of contact to troubleshoot problems should always be provided.

Clinical research evidence

There are over 750 hits for the MeSH term 'transcutaneous electric nerve stimulation' with limits 'randomised controlled trial' in

Table 18.1 Systematic review evidence.

Condition	Reference	Sample	Reviewers' conclusion
Acute Pain			
Acute pain	Walsh et al., 2009	12 RCTs (919 patients) on TENS	Evidence inconclusive
Post-operative pain	Carroll et al., 1996	17 RCTs (786 patients) on TENS	Evidence of no effect
Post-throacotomy pain	Freynet and Falcoz, 2010	9 RCTs (645 patients) on TENS	Evidence of effect as an adjuvant
Post-operative analgesic consumption	Bjordal et al., 2003	21 RCTs (964 patients) on TENS	Evidence of effect
Labour pain	Carroll et al., 1997	10 RCTs (877 women) on TENS	Evidence of no effect
Labour pain	Dowswell et al., 2009	19 RCTs (1671 women) on TENS	Evidence inconclusive
Primary dysmenorrhoea	Proctor et al., 2003	7 RCTs (213 patients) on TENS	Evidence of effect
Chronic Pain			
Chronic pain	Carroll et al., 2001	19 RCTs (652 patients) on TENS	Evidence inconclusive
Chronic pain (an update of Carroll et al., 2001)	Nnoaham and Kumbang, 2008	25 RCTs (1281 patients) on TENS	Evidence inconclusive
Low back pain	Khadilkar et al., 2008	3 RCTs (197 patients) on TENS	Evidence inconclusive
Low back pain	Poitras et al., 2008	6 RCTs (375 patients) on TENS	Evidence of effect
Low back pain	Dubinsky and Myasaki, 2010	2 RCTs (201 patients) on TENS	Evidence of no effect
Osteoarthritic knee pain	Bjordal et al., 2007	36 RCTs (2434 patients) of physical agents with 7 RCTs (414 patients) on TENS using adequate technique	Evidence of effect
Osteoarthritic knee pain	Rutjes et al., 2009	18 RCTs (275 patients) on TENS	Evidence inconclusive
Rheumatoid arthritis of the hand	Brosseau et al., 2003	3 RCT (78 patients) on TENS	Evidence of effect
Chronic musculoskeletal pain	Johnson and Martinson, 2007	38 RCTs (1227 patients) of any electrical nerve stimulation with 32 RCTs on TENS	Evidence of effect
Neuropathic pain	Crucci et al., 2007	9 RCTs (200 patients) on TENS	Evidence of effect
Painful diabetic neuropathy	Jin et al., 2010	3 RCTs (78 patients) on TENS	Evidence of effect
Painful diabetic neuropathy	Dubinksy and Miyasaki, 2010	2 RCTs (55 patients) on TENS	Evidence of effect
Chronic recurrent headache	Bronfort et al., 2004	22 RCTs (2628 patients) of physical agents but no RCTs on TENS	Lack of available evidence
Post-stroke shoulder pain	Price and Pandyan, 2001	4 RCTs (170 patients) of any surface electrical stimulation with 2 RCTs on TENS	Evidence inconclusive
Whiplash and mechanical neck disorders	Kroeling et al., 2009	18 RCTs (1043 patients) of any electrotherapy with 7 RCTs (88 patients) on TENS	Evidence of effect
Cancer pain	Robb et al., 2009	2 RCTs (64 patients) on TENS	Evidence inconclusive
Phantom limb and Stump pain	Mulvey et al., 2010	0 RCTs	No evidence available

PubMed [as of 16 March 2011]. Many randomised controlled trials (RCTs) have methodological shortcomings including inadequate TENS technique and this has hindered definitive conclusions about effectiveness.

TENS and acute pain

TENS is of limited benefit as a stand-alone treatment for severe to moderate pain, although a Cochrane review on TENS as an isolated treatment for acute pain in adults was inconclusive due to insufficient extractable data. Opinion is divided about effectiveness in combination with pharmacotherapy in the acute pain setting (Table 18.1). Early systematic reviews on post-operative pain reported negative outcomes. Recent systematic reviews have found that TENS was ineffective as a stand-alone therapy for severe post-thoracotomy pain, but useful as an adjunct to analgesics for moderate post-thoracotomy pain and for reducing post-operative analgesic consumption. A Cochrane review on TENS for labour pain was inconclusive and a meta-analysis found that TENS was superior to sham TENS for primary dysmenorrhoea pain. RCTs on TENS for acute orofacial pain, painful dental procedures, fractured ribs, acute lower back pain and angina suggest that TENS is superior to sham TENS.

TENS and chronic pain

The most recent Cochrane review on TENS for non-malignant chronic pain was inconclusive. Systematic reviews on TENS for chronic low back pain have been positive, negative or inconclusive. Meta-analyses on TENS for osteoarthritic knee pain have been positive and inconclusive. A large meta-analysis found TENS to be superior to placebo TENS for chronic musculoskeletal pain and smaller meta-analyses have found TENS superior to placebo TENS for neck pain, rheumatoid arthritis of the hand, chronic recurrent headache and peripheral diabetic neuropathy. The European Federation of Neurological Societies (EFNS) Task Force for neurostimulation therapy for neuropathic pain found that TENS was superior to placebo based on nine controlled trials with data extracted for 200 patients. Most systematic reviews are inconclusive (e.g. post-stroke shoulder pain, cancer pain, post-amputee pain).

At present, guidelines from the National Institute of Health and Clinical Excellence (NICE) (www.nice.org.uk) in the United Kingdom recommend that TENS should not be offered for early management of persistent non-specific low back pain or for women in established labour, although it may be beneficial in early stages of labour. NICE recommends that TENS should be offered as an adjunct for short-term relief of osteoarthritic knee pain and for rheumatoid arthritis of the hand.

References

Bjordal, JM, Johnson, MI & Ljunggreen, AE (2003) Transcutaneous electrical nerve stimulation (TENS) can reduce postoperative analgesic consumption. A meta-analysis with assessment of optimal treatment parameters for postoperative pain. *Eur J Pain*, **7** (2), 181–188.

Bjordal, JM, Johnson, MI, Lopes-Martins, RA, Bogen, B, Chow, R & Ljunggren, AE (2007) Short-term efficacy of physical interventions in osteoarthritic knee pain. A systematic review and meta-analysis of randomised placebo-controlled trials. *BMC Musculoskelet Disord*, **8**, 51.

Bronfort G, Nilsson, N, Haas, M, Evans, R, Goldsmith, CH, Assendelft, WJ & Bouter, LM (2004) Non-invasive physical treatments for chronic/recurrent headache. *Cochrane Database of Systematic Reviews* 3 (Art. No.: CD001878). doi: 10.1002/14651858.CD001878.pub2.

Brosseau, L, Yonge, KA, Robinson, V, Marchand, S, Judd, M, Wells, G & Tugwell, P (2003) Transcutaneous electrical nerve stimulation (TENS) for the treatment of rheumatoid arthritis in the hand. *Cochrane Database of Systematic Reviews* 3 (Art. No.: CD004377). doi: 10.1002/14651858. CD004377.

Carroll, D, Moore, RA, McQuay, HJ, Fairman, F, Tramer, M & Leijon, G (2001) Transcutaneous electrical nerve stimulation (TENS) for chronic pain. *Cochrane Database Syst Rev* (**3**): CD003222.

Carroll, D, Tramer, M, McQuay, H, Nye, B & Moore, A (1996) Randomization is important in studies with pain outcomes: systematic review of transcutaneous electrical nerve stimulation in acute postoperative pain. *Br J Anaesth*, **77** (6), 798–803.

Carroll, D, Tramer, M, McQuay, H, Nye, B & Moore, A (1997) Transcutaneous electrical nerve stimulation in labour pain: a systematic review. *Br J Obstet Gynaecol*, **104** (2), 169–175.

Cruccu, G, Aziz, TZ, Garcia-Larrea, L, Hansson, P, Jensen, TS, Lefaucheur, JP, *et al.* (2007) EFNS guidelines on neurostimulation therapy for neuropathic pain. *Eur J Neurol*, **14** (9), 952–970.

Dowswell, T, Bedwell, C, Lavender, T & Neilson, JP (2009) Transcutaneous electrical nerve stimulation (TENS) for pain relief in labour. *Cochrane Database of Systematic Reviews* 2 (Art. No.: CD007214). doi: 10.1002/14651858.CD007214.pub2.

Dubinsky, RM & Miyasaki, J (2010) Assessment: efficacy of transcutaneous electric nerve stimulation in the treatment of pain in neurologic disorders (an evidence-based review): report of the Therapeutics and Technology Assessment Subcommittee of the American Academy of Neurology. *Neurology*, **74** (2), 173–176.

Freynet, A & Falcoz, PE (2010) Is transcutaneous electrical nerve stimulation effective in relieving postoperative pain after thoracotomy? *Interact Cardiovasc Thorac Surg*, **10** (2), 283–288.

Jin, DM, Xu, Y, Geng, DF & Yan, TB (2010) Effect of transcutaneous electrical nerve stimulation on symptomatic diabetic peripheral neuropathy: a meta-analysis of randomized controlled trials. *Diabetes Res Clin Pract*, **89** (1), 10–15.

Johnson, MI (2001) Transcutaneous Electrical Nerve Stimulation (TENS) and TENS-like devices. Do they provide pain relief? *Pain Reviews*, **8**, 121–128.

Johnson, M & Martinson, M (2007) Efficacy of electrical nerve stimulation for chronic musculoskeletal pain: a meta-analysis of randomized controlled trials. *Pain*, **130** (1–2), 157–165.

Khadilkar, A, Odebiyi, DO, Brosseau, L & Wells, GA (2008) Transcutaneous electrical nerve stimulation (TENS) versus placebo for chronic low-back pain. *Cochrane Database of Systematic Reviews* 4 (Art. No.: CD003008). doi: 10.1002/14651858.CD003008.pub3.

Kroeling, P, Gross, A, Goldsmith, CH, Burnie, SJ, Haines, T, Graham, N & Brant, A (2009) Electrotherapy for neck pain. *Cochrane Database of Systematic Reviews* 4 (Art. No.: CD004251). doi: 10.1002/14651858.CD004251.pub4.

Mulvey, MR, Bagnall, A-M, Johnson, MI & Marchant, PR (2010) Transcutaneous electrical nerve stimulation (TENS) for phantom pain and stump pain following amputation in adults. *Cochrane Database of Systematic Reviews* 5 (Art. No.: CD007264). doi: 10.1002/14651858.CD007264.pub2.

Nnoaham, KE & Kumbang, J (2008) Transcutaneous electrical nerve stimulation (TENS) for chronic pain. *Cochrane Database of Systematic Reviews* 3 (Art. No.: CD003222). doi: 10.1002/14651858.CD003222.pub2.

Poitras, S & Brosseau, L (2008) Evidence-informed management of chronic low back pain with transcutaneous electrical nerve stimulation, interferential current, electrical muscle stimulation, ultrasound, and thermotherapy. *Spine J*, **8** (1), 226–233.

Price, CI & Pandyan, AD (2001) Electrical stimulation for preventing and treating post-stroke shoulder pain: a systematic Cochrane review. *Clin Rehabil*, **15** (1), 5–19.

Proctor, ML, Farquhar, CM, Stones, RW, He, L, Zhu, X & Brown, J (2003) Transcutaneous electrical nerve stimulation and acupuncture for primary dysmenorrhoea. *Cochrane Database of Systematic Reviews* 1 (Art. No.: CD002123). doi: 10.1002/14651858.CD002123.

Robb, K, Oxberry, SG, Bennett, MI, Johnson, MI, Simpson, KH & Searle, RD (2009) A Cochrane systematic review of transcutaneous electrical nerve stimulation for cancer pain. *J Pain Symptom Manage*, **37** (4), 746–753.

Rutjes, AW, Nuesch, E, Sterchi, R, Kalichman, L, Hendriks, E, Osiri, M, *et al.* (2009) Transcutaneous electrostimulation for osteoarthritis of the knee. *Cochrane Database of Systematic Reviews* 4 (Art. No.: CD002823). doi: 10.1002/14651858.CD002823.pub2.

Walsh, DM, Howe, TE, Johnson, MI, Moran, F & Sluka, KA (2009) Transcutaneous electrical nerve stimulation for acute pain. *Cochrane Database of Systematic Reviews* 2 (Art. No.: CD006142). doi: 10.1002/14651858.CD006142.pub2.

Further reading

Barlas, P & Lundeberg, T (2006) Transcutaneous electrical nerve stimulation and acupuncture. In: McMahon, S & Koltzenburg, M (eds) *Melzack and Wall's Textbook of Pain*, 5th edn. Philadelphia, PA: Elsevier Churchill Livingstone. pp. 583–590.

DeSantana, JM, Walsh, DM, Vance, C, Rakel, BA & Sluka, KA (2008) Effectiveness of transcutaneous electrical nerve stimulation for treatment of hyperalgesia and pain. *Curr Rheumatol Rep*, **10** (6), 492–499.

Johnson, MI (2008) Transcutaneous Electrical Nerve Stimulation. In: Watson, T (ed.) *Electrotherapy: Evidence based practice*. New York: Churchill Livingstone. pp. 253–296.

Johnson, MI & Bjrodal, JM (2011) Transcutaneous Electrical Nerve Stimulation for the management of painful conditions: focus on neuropathic pain. *Expert Reviews in Neurotherapeutics*, **11** (5), 735–753.

Johnson, MI & Walsh, DM (2010) Pain: continued uncertainty of TENS' effectiveness for pain relief. *Nat Rev Rheumatol*, **6** (6), 314–316.

Walsh, D (1997) *TENS. Clinical applications and related theory*, 1st edn. New York: Churchill Livingstone.

CHAPTER 19

Complementary and Alternative Strategies

Margaret Cullen and Fiona MacPherson

Western General Hospital, Edinburgh, UK

OVERVIEW

- This chapter briefly reviews the place of three complementary and alternative therapies in the management of acute and chronic pain

- Acupuncture may be helpful in selected acute and chronic pain conditions

- Hypnosis is most commonly used as a self-management technique in chronic pain

- Aromatherapy may be useful to promote relaxation and treat painful joint and muscular conditions

- There are significant resource implications in delivering complementary and alternative therapies for pain over the longer term

---

Introduction

The use of complementary and alternative therapies in the management of pain pre-dates many of the more conventional therapies described in this book. Nevertheless, their use within health services remains relatively limited due both to some scepticism regarding their effectiveness and to limited availability of healthcare resources. Space is too limited to debate the efficacy of these treatments. Therefore, this chapter concentrates on a brief overview of the aims, techniques and availability of three treatments–acupuncture, hypnotherapy and aromatherapy.

Who should deliver the treatment?

A variety of healthcare professionals may deliver these treatments and in some areas volunteers may also be involved. Regulation of those delivering complementary and alternative therapies remains rather problematic. There are guidelines from different healthcare providers on the delivery of complementary and alternative therapies and these should be consulted where they exist. Clearly, healthcare professionals must adhere to all requirements set out by their own statutory regulatory bodies and, in addition, must receive

appropriate training in their particular therapy and must abide by the standards and guidelines of the association or regulatory body that oversees that therapy. Websites (with extensive additional information for both professionals and patients) for some of the relevant professional associations and the disciplines they represent are in Box 19.1.

Box 19.1 **Useful resources for professional associations involved with delivery of acupuncture, hypnosis and aromatherapy**

www.aacp.org.uk Acupuncture Association of Chartered Physiotherapists (chartered physiotherapists)
www.medical-acupuncture.co.uk British Medical Acupuncture Society (Regulated healthcare practitioners including doctors and dentists who practice acupuncture)
www.bscah.com British Society of Clinical and Academic Hypnosis (Medical and dental practitioners, psychologists and other health professionals)
www.bsmdhscotland.com British Society of Medical and Dental Hypnosis (Scotland) (Medical and dental practitioners)
www.ifparoma.org International Federation of Professional Aromatherapists (Regulated healthcare practitioners and others trained in aromatherapy)
(All sites accessed 10 December 2011)

As with any other medical intervention, patients receiving any complementary or alternative therapy must receive a full explanation of what is involved and give formal consent. The therapist must keep an accurate record of all treatments and outcomes. Within the pain clinic context these notes are usually kept as part of the multidisciplinary record.

Acupuncture

In pain management services most acupuncture treatment is delivered by healthcare professionals (usually doctors, nurses or physiotherapists) who have additional training in acupuncture techniques but who work within the diagnostic and management parameters of conventional Western medicine, using needling techniques based on conventional understanding of the neurophysiology of pain.

ABC of Pain, First edition. Edited by Lesley A Colvin and Marie Fallon.
© 2012 Blackwell Publishing Ltd. Published 2012 by Blackwell Publishing Ltd.

This contrasts with practitioners of Traditional Chinese Medicine, who use acupuncture techniques based on an ancient complex Chinese philosophical system that envisages 'Qi' or energy running through meridians and a requirement to balance Yin and Yang (Figure 19.1).

Acupuncture is probably the commonest complementary therapy offered in chronic pain clinics. In addition, it is widely available from physiotherapists for the management of more acute musculoskeletal pains, usually to allow the patient to engage more fully with other physiotherapy interventions. On a more intermittent basis, acupuncture is also provided in primary care by a small number of enthusiastic general practitioners and some nurses.

As with any other therapeutic intervention, acupuncture for pain management should be delivered after appropriate investigations have been carried out and a diagnosis made (even if this is simply a diagnosis of exclusion). Patients are typically offered a trial block of 3 to 6 weekly treatments in the first instance. Side effects are usually minimal and may include fatigue, bruising, rarely allergy to the needles and occasionally a worsening of symptomatology. Modern acupuncture needles are single use and pre-sterilised, as with any other medical needle (Figure 19.2). Needles are 'stimulated' either

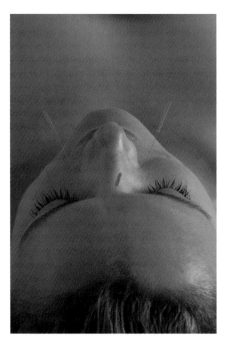

Figure 19.3 Facial acupuncture. (Photograph by permission of the British Medical Acupuncture Society).

by manual rotation by the therapist or by electro-acupuncture. Depth of insertion depends on both the type of needling chosen and, more importantly, the anatomy of the area to be treated. Serious adverse events reported after acupuncture are rare but include cardiac tamponade and pneumothorax.

Patients with a variety of musculoskeletal pains, including low back pain, neck pain and osteo-arthritic knee pain, are all suitable candidates for a trial of acupuncture. Patients with chronic headache and facial pain may also respond well (Figure 19.3). Significant needle phobia, known allergy to needles and infection in the area to be treated are all contraindications to treatment. Anticoagulant therapy is not an absolute contraindication as long as extra consideration is given to anatomical considerations and depth of needling.

Acupuncture may provide symptomatic benefit in chronic pain conditions but is not curative. Repeat 'top-up' acupuncture treatments are required over time. The main restriction to these 'top-ups' in pain clinics is limited availability of resources. Different clinics manage the problem in a variety of ways. It is the author's practice to offer a small number of further treatments only to the patients who have shown the most significant and prolonged response to the initial block of treatments. Patients may seek other treatment providers, for example via the British Medical Acupuncture Society, or occasionally interested general practitioners will take over their long-term treatment – though similar resource constraints apply in general practice.

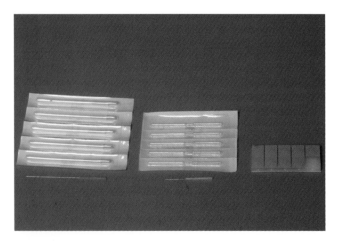

Figure 19.1 Traditional Chinese needles now used for teaching purposes only.

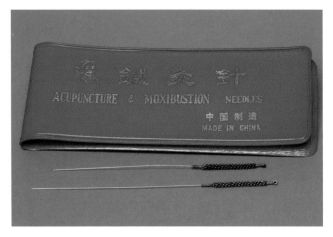

Figure 19.2 A range of modern acupuncture needles. (Photograph by permission of the British Medical Acupuncture Society).

Hypnosis

Hypnosis has been used in the management of acute pain in a variety of situations, including dentistry, burns dressing changes, labour and invasive medical procedures. However, it is more commonly employed in the management of chronic pain because, to be fully effective, the technique must be taught, modified if necessary, practised regularly and, ideally, become second nature to the patient.

The aims of hypnosis in chronic pain are surprisingly similar in some respects to those of pain management programmes. Both aim to de-medicalise the chronic pain condition and encourage a sense of self-efficacy with associated improvement in mood as confidence grows. Patients suitable for hypnosis are those who are comfortable with the concept and prepared to work at the technique. Some studies suggest better outcomes for patients with high levels of hypnotic suggestibility. A number of scores exist to measure this, if wished, before instituting treatment. Patients with severe depression or psychosis are not usually considered suitable for hypnotic techniques.

Treatments involve a number of sessions where the patient is taught to self-hypnotise and to use visualisation, or other methods, to reduce the level of their pain (Boxes 19.2 and 19.3). It is stressed to the patient that the technique is thereafter 'owned' by them and that regular practice will improve both their competence and confidence.

Box 19.2 **Elements of a typical hypnosis session**

- Induction of hypnosis
- Deepening
- Rehearsal of the selected method of pain management (Box 19.3)
- Ego-strengthening
- Post-hypnotic suggestion
- Emergence

Box 19.3 **Some hypnotic visualisations and suggestions that may be used for pain management**

- Use of imagery, for example use of a pain dial – visualising actively turning the pain numbers down or changing the visualised 'colours' of a particular pain
- Suggestions of numbness and lack of sensation in the painful area
- Reinterpretation of symptoms, for example a sensation of pleasant warmth rather than pain
- Displacement of symptoms, for example suggesting that the pain is only experienced in the toes rather than the whole leg

---

Patients may initially have significant misconceptions about the nature of medical hypnosis. It is important, therefore, to explain that the 'trance' of medical hypnosis is not deep. It has been likened to the level of consciousness of a person who is deeply engrossed in an activity such as reading a book, listening to music or daydreaming. The subject remains dimly aware of their surroundings and can return to full consciousness at any time should they wish.

Patients usually attend for a few sessions. Over time the technique or visualisation for pain management may be modified depending on how effective the patient finds it. A recording of the session is made and the patient is encouraged to practice daily. However, the ultimate aim (not achievable for every patient) is for them to gain enough confidence to dispense with the tape and become completely self-sufficient. Not all patients may be able to control their pain using the techniques described for pain management. However, many still gain benefit from the deep relaxation experienced during a session of self-hypnosis.

Doctors or psychologists usually deliver hypnosis in the pain clinic setting. Since there is strong emphasis on teaching the patient a self-management technique with no long-term requirement for regular follow-up, there are fewer resource implications than with other complementary or alternative therapies.

Aromatherapy massage

Increasingly, aromatherapy massage has gained in popularity with the public and health professionals. It is now widely accepted as a complement to conventional medicine and is offered in a small number of pain clinics. In chronic pain the patient is encouraged to self-manage and incorporate various techniques in a bid to manage the pain, increase function and improve quality of life. Aromatherapy massage may be one component in a planned treatment programme.

Aromatherapy is the controlled use of essential oils to enhance and promote the health of the individual. The oils are highly concentrated essences and are extracted from flowers, leaves, bark, twigs, roots and the fruits from plants (Figure 19.4). An essential oil may have hundreds of individual chemical components, most of which have their own characteristic smell and therapeutic properties, including relaxing, stimulating, anti-inflammatory, analgesic and promoting circulation. When used appropriately they have the ability to affect emotions and relieve many physical ailments (Tables 19.1 and 19.2).

It is thought they work directly on the limbic system in the brain (the area that controls our emotions) and block pain transmission by creating a counter-irritant stimulus. The essential oils can be used in a variety of ways, in the bath or shower, inhalation, application

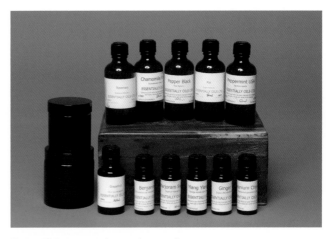

Figure 19.4 A range of aromatherapy oils.

Table 19.1 Common conditions treated with aromatherapy massage and a selection of oils used in their management (the list is not exhaustive).

Condition	Oil
Anxiety	Roman Chamomile, lavender, geranium, bergamot
Insomnia	Chamomiles, lavender, marjoram, rose, ylangylang
Stress and tension	Bergamot, lavender, geranium, grapefruit, marjoram, rosemary, ylangylang
Muscle spasm	Marjoram, ginger, black pepper, peppermint, plai
Joint pain	Eucalyptus, chamomiles, plai, peppermint, black pepper

Table 19.2 Selection of oils and the main chemical constituents.

Common name	Main chemical constituents	Contraindications
Roman Chamomile	Principally esters of angelic acid (85%), tiglic acid, pinene, farnesol, chamazulene, pinocarvone and cineol	None Non-toxic and non-irritant (up to 4%)
Lavender	Linalyl acetate (40%), linalool, lavandulol, terpineol, cineol and caryophyllene	None Non-toxic and non-irritant
Black Pepper	Monoterpenes (70–80%), myrcene, sabinene, careen, sesquiterpenes, caryophyllene and bisabolene	None Non-toxic and non-irritant in low dilution
Grapefruit	Limonene (90%), paradisiol, citronellal, assorted esters and coumarins	None Non-toxic and non-irritant

of compresses or creams and probably most frequently through massage.

Massage therapy involves applying pressure with stroking and kneading movements to different parts of the body to aid relaxation by increasing blood flow and reducing muscle tension; it provides temporary analgesia by activating the 'pain gate' mechanism of pain. When used in combination with each other, the massage aids the penetration of the oils and creates an arena for relaxation both mentally and physically. For massage purposes a blend of essential oils in a carrier such as grapeseed oil is tailored to the individual. The main functions of the carrier oil areas a diluent for the fat-soluble essential oil and as lubrication. Most blends will contain anything from one to four oils in a 1–5% dilution depending on the condition of the patient.

Pregnancy is not an absolute contradiction but aromatherapy massage should probably be offered after the first trimester and it is important that the therapist is aware of any other medical conditions, such as high blood pressure.

In the author's practice the patient is offered four weekly treatments and is encouraged to bring a family member or friend for instruction in the massage and the use of oils. This allows the patient to try the treatment in a safe environment and to decide if

Table 19.3 Record of therapeutic response to a 4-week course of aromatherapy. Pain scores are recorded on a scale of 0–10, with 10 being the worst pain possible.

	Pre-massage pain score	Post-massage pain score
Week 1	9	5
Week 2	9	3
Week 3	9	4
Week 4	6	3

the therapy is beneficial. If benefit is obtained, the patient is then able to continue the treatments at home rather than depend on the limited treatment resources of the average pain clinic. Table 19.3 shows typical results from a successful course of treatments with gradual improvement over time.

Evidence-based summary

- Clear evidence for the efficacy of complementary and alternative therapies in the management of pain tends to be limited.
- Hypnotic techniques are beneficial for some types of acute pain and are useful in the management of chronic pain in the context of a multidisciplinary management approach.
- Acupuncture is effective in the management of some acute pain problems and is probably beneficial for longer periods in selected patients with chronic pain.
- Aromatherapy massage aids relaxation and improves pain management in some acute and chronic pain conditions.

Further reading

Baldry, PE (2004) *Acupuncture, Trigger Points and Musculoskeletal Pain.* Edinburgh: Churchill Livingstone, 2004.

Chang, M-Y, Wang, S-Y & Chen, C-H (2002) Effects of massage on pain and anxiety during labour: a randomised controlled trial in Taiwan. *Journal of Advanced Nursing,* **38** (1), 68–73

Filshie, J & White, A (1998) *Medical Acupuncture: A Western Scientific Approach* Edinburgh: Churchill Livingstone.

Heap, M & Aravind, KK (2002) *Hartland's Medical and Dental Hypnosis.* Edinburgh: Churchill Livingstone.

Kessler, RS, Patterson, DR, Dane, J (2003) Hypnosis and relaxation with pain patients: Evidence for effectiveness. *Seminars in Pain Medicine, 1* (2), 67–78.

Manheimer, E, Linde, K, Lao, L, Bouter, LM & Berman, BM (2007) Meta-analysis: acupuncture for osteoarthritis of the knee. *Ann Intern Med,* **146** (12), 868–877.

National Institute for Health and Clinical Excellence (2009) *NICE guideline on low back pain: early management of persistent non-specific low back pain.* Available at http://guidance.nice.org.uk/CG88 (accessed on 26 October 2010).

Price, S & Price, L (1995) *Aromatherapy for Health Professionals.* New York: Churchill Livingstone.

Saeki, Y & Shiohara, M (2001) Physiological Effects of Inhaling Fragrances. *The International Journal of Aromatherapy,* **11** (3), 116–125.

Stux, G, Berman, B & Pomeranz, B (2003) *Basics of Acupuncture.* Springer.

CHAPTER 20

Opioids in Chronic Non-malignant Pain

Eija Kalso

University of Helsinki/Pain Clinic, Helsinki University Central Hospital, Helsinki, Finland

OVERVIEW

- Opioids in chronic non-malignant pain can be considered if other usual methods do not provide enough pain relief or are contraindicated

- Patients show significant variation in opioid response, which should be assessed during a 1–2 month trial period and monitored carefully thereafter

- Opioid therapy should relieve pain and improve function and quality of life and can be useful in both nociceptive and neuropathic pain treatment

- The prescribing physician should be familiar with the patient's psychosocial status; an opioid contract clarifying the patient's rights and responsibilities may be useful in some circumstances

- Controlled-release opioids should be used in preference to rapid onset short-acting opioids

- Opioid therapy should not be considered as a life-long option when managing non-malignant pain

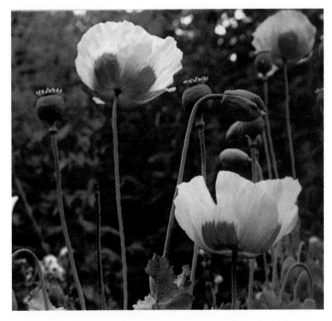

Figure 20.1 Opium that is derived from the poppy, *Papaver somniferum*, has been used in pain relief for millenia.

Background

Opioids are the oldest (Figure 20.1) and the most important analgesics in the management of acute and cancer pain but their use is more controversial and challenging in chronic non-malignant pain. Opioids can be effective and safe also in chronic non-malignant pain if they are used wisely, with a thorough understanding of the patient and the pharmacology of opioids.

Recent advances in pharmacogenetics have increased our understanding of why opioid responses vary so much between individuals and conditions. Opioids often cause adverse effects that can be serious. This chapter discusses the use of opioids in chronic pain. It provides information about the efficacy of opioids in different chronic pain conditions, guidelines that have been introduced to help the clinician in patient selection and follow-up, and the pharmacokinetic and pharmacogenetic differences of opioids.

ABC of Pain, First edition. Edited by Lesley A Colvin and Marie Fallon.
© 2012 Blackwell Publishing Ltd. Published 2012 by Blackwell Publishing Ltd.

The endogenous opioid system

Opioid receptors and their endogenous ligands modulate numerous physiological functions, such as nociception, mood, reward, learning, stress response, hormonal functions, appetite, sleep, immune function and gastrointestinal function. Three receptor classes – mu (MOR), delta (DOR) and kappa (KOR) – have been described by pharmacological approaches. More recently, using cloning techniques, an additional type of opioid receptor has been found – the ORL1 (orphanin receptor like) or NOP (nociceptin) receptor. MOR is the major molecular target for morphine. Opioid receptors have a wide range of functions, some of which are outlined in Figure 20.2.

Opioid receptors are located throughout the central and peripheral nervous system. Opioid receptors in the dorsal horn of the spinal cord have an important role in the modulation of pain. Opioid receptors in the brain stem are involved in the regulation of arousal, respiration and both anti- and pro-nociceptive effects. Opioid receptors are found almost everywhere in the cerebrum and

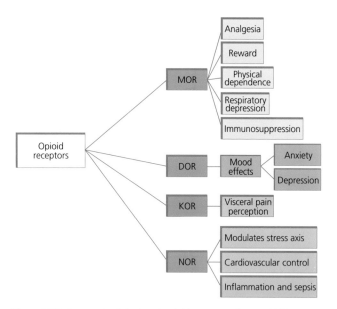

Figure 20.2 Some potential roles of opioid receptor subtypes. MOR = mu opioid receptor; DOR = delta opioid receptor; KOR = kappa opioid receptor; NOR = nocieptin/orphanin FQ peptide opioid receptor.

cerebellum. In the periphery, opioids are involved in the regulation of gastrointestinal function. Activation of MORs in the gut leads to increased absorption of water from the stools and spasticity of the gut. Peripheral opioid receptors are involved in the regulation of inflammation and the immune system.

Opioids for chronic non-cancer pain: what is the evidence for efficacy?

Several systematic reviews have indicated moderate short-term efficacy (up to 3 months) of opioids in both osteoarthritis-related and neuropathic pain. Both weak and strong opioids were better than placebo for pain. Mean pain relief with strong opioids in these studies was about 30% in both neuropathic and osteoarthritic pain when mean daily doses of 40 mg of oxycodone or 80–100 mg of morphine were used. The effect size for improved function has, however, been small. Variation in response between patients has been considerable and the placebo response has been quite significant. Musculoskeletal pains other than osteoarthritis have not shown long-term benefit from opioids. Opioids may be efficacious for short-term pain relief for back pain whereas their long-term efficacy is unclear.

Aberrant medication-taking behaviour has been reported to occur in up to one in four back pain patients. Continuous opioid therapy is rarely advisable for refractory chronic daily headache because of limited efficacy. There are no controlled trials on the efficacy and safety of opioids in visceral pain or fibromyalgia.

Opioids should be used only if there has been a comprehensive assessment that indicates potential efficacy. Guidance for the initiation of treatment with strong opioids and requirements for successful therapy with opioids are given in Boxes 20.1 and 20.2, respectively.

Box 20.1 Initiating treatment with strong opioids

Opioid therapy can be introduced by the GP if:

- the cause of the pain is known
- the pain is likely to respond to opioids
- opioids are needed for a restricted period only
- the patient does not have any major psychosocial problems
- the patient does not have a history of drug or alcohol abuse

The patient should be evaluated for opioid therapy at a multidisciplinary pain clinic if:

- the cause of the pain problem is not clear
- the patient is young
- opioid therapy is expected to last for a prolonged period (several months)
- the patient has major psychosocial problems
- the patient has a history of drug or alcohol abuse

Box 20.2 Requirements for successful therapy with opioids

Opioid therapy is likely to be successful if the prescribing physician:

- has adequate knowledge of opioid pharmacology
- considers carefully the benefits and harms of opioid therapy
- takes responsibility for the follow-up of opioid therapy and takes careful records
- is willing to consult a pain specialist when needed
- does not increase the opioid dose without careful consideration
- titrates down opioid therapy if the patient does not receive significant benefit from it

Opioid therapy is likely to be successful if the patient:

- has been informed of the potential benefits and harms of opioid therapy
- is willing to follow instructions regarding opioid therapy
- is willing to actively pursue other methods of pain relief (physical activity, pain management groups)
- is willing to provide a urine test for opioid screening if considered necessary

Risks and benefits of opioid therapy

The biggest difficulty in the long-term management of chronic pain with opioids is risk-benefit analysis (Figure 20.3). Some risks are common and are usually easy to prevent (e.g. constipation) whereas others (e.g. opioid addiction) are rare, difficult to predict and to treat. Several risk assessment tools have been developed for opioid misuse by chronic pain patients. Some pain clinics use an opioid contract (Box 20.3) and urine screening.

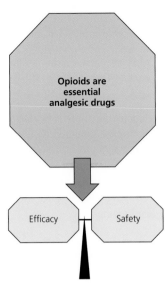

Figure 20.3 Titrating the dose – balancing between analgesia and adverse effects – is the challenge for managing pain with opioids.

Table 20.1 Treating pain with strong opioids: differences between malignant and non-malignant pain.

	Malignant pain	**Non-malignant pain**
Primary endpoint	Alleviation of pain and suffering	Pain relief and improvement of function
Initiation of opioid therapy	Every physician's duty	Usually by a multidisciplinary pain clinic
Opioid dependence	Not a problem	Should be considered as a potential problem
Treating breakthrough pain with short-acting opioids	Part of good practice	Not routinely
Invasive methods of administration	When indicated	Extremely rarely (e.g. subarachnoid or epidural)
Opioid adverse effects	Should not prevent opioid therapy; adverse effects vigorously treated	Often lead to patient stopping opioid therapy despite treatment of adverse effects.

Box 20.3 **Features of an opioid contract**

A contract in opioid therapy should include at least the following aspects:

- Description of opioid therapy including possible benefits and harms
- The patient is obliged to inform the physician or the team if he/she uses other analgesics or psychotropic drugs
- The patient should not ask another physician to prescribe analgesics
- The prescribed opioid should be taken as advised by the physician and opioids should never be given to another person
- Opioids should be kept in a locked place and special care should be taken to avoid children having access to them. The police should be informed if opioids are stolen
- Opioids can decrease psychomotor function even though tolerance to a stable dose usually develops within 2–3 weeks. Dose increases, additional doses, other psychotropic drugs, sedatives and opioids decrease the psychomotor function further. These facts need to be considered if the patient needs to be capable of operating machines or driving a car
- The patient needs a document (either from the physician or the pharmacy) indicating the medical need for the opioid prescription when travelling abroad. The amount of opioids allowed for personal use is limited

---

There is some evidence to suggest that combining CBT with long-term opioid therapy may improve analgesia and reduce dose escalation. Both long duration of therapy and high opioid doses are related to more adverse effects.

Most opioid adverse effects are dose-related (e.g. hormonal effects). Tolerance develops to some adverse effects (e.g. sedation) whereas no tolerance seems to develop to constipation.

Guidelines regarding the role of opioids in the treatment of various chronic painful conditions or chronic opioid treatment in general have been published. They have been written by expert panels that have used the evidence available. It is important to note that opioids are not a first line medication in any of these chronic pain conditions. The opioid treatment protocols that are used in cancer pain are not applicable directly to non-malignant pain (Table 20.1).

Codeine and tramadol are considered weak opioids and both are pro-drugs regarding opioid activity, that is the drugs themselves are inactive until metabolised to active drug. Buprenorphine is a more potent opioid. The 'strong opioids' that are in clinical use in the United Kingdom include morphine, oxycodone, hydromorphone and methadone. Methadone should be prescribed only by physicians who have special competence in opioid pharmacology.

Basic pharmacology of opioids: relevance for clinical use

Tramadol itself has only weak affinity to the MOR. Opioid analgesia is mediated by the M1 (O-desmethyltramadol) metabolite that has a 200-fold greater affinity to the MOR than the parent compound. Tramadol also inhibits the reuptake of norepinephrine and releases serotonin. These effects are important for the efficacy of tramadol in the management of neuropathic pain.

Tapentadol is a new MOR agonist that has a 50 times lower affinity to the MOR than morphine. Tapentadol has a dual action in analgesia as it also inhibits the reuptake of norepinephrine. This dual action may explain the good efficacy of tapentadol compared with 'strong opioids' in the management of low back pain and pain due to osteoarthritis. The gastrointestinal safety seems to be better with tapentadol compared with strong opioids. Open label studies indicate that tapentadol may be effective in diabetic peripheral neuropathic pain. It is not a pro-drug and it is not susceptible to CYP-mediated drug interactions.

Morphine, oxycodone, methadone and fentanyl are all MOR agonists in doses that are commonly used to treat pain in the clinic. Differences, however, exist between these opioids in their capacity to activate the MORs.

Some opioids have non-opioid effects that are relevant for their analgesic profile. Racemic methadone consists of two enantiomers (l- and d-) both of which have been described to be non-competitive N-methyl-D-aspartate (NMDA)-receptor antagonists. It is l-methadone that is responsible for the MOR effects, while d-methadone is only a weak opioid agonist.

Pharmacokinetic aspects and potential for drug interactions

Rate of onset of action

Pharmaceutical technology has developed oral sustained or modified-release formulations that provide stable plasma concentrations with once or twice daily oral dosing. Such formulations have been developed for morphine, oxycodone, hydromorphone tapentadol and tramadol. Usually the time to maximum plasma drug concentration (T_{max}) is 2–4 hours. Normal or immediate-release formulations with a T_{max} of 30–60 min are used if faster onset is needed.

Transdermal

Transdermal administration has been developed to achieve slow onset with stable concentrations, nearly 3 days for fentanyl and 7 days for buprenorphine. Transdermal administration requires a lipophilic opioid. Any factors that increase skin perfusion (fever, sauna) will increase absorption, whereas this is decreased if skin perfusion is reduced (cachexia, hypovolaemia or vasoconstriction). The first-pass metabolism is usually high for lipophilic opioids, and consequently oral bioavailability is very low (Table 20.2), such that they cannot be taken orally.

Pharmacokinetic properties

The main pharmacokinetic parameters of some commonly used opioids are shown in Table 20.2. The clearance of most opioids is high, and hepatic blood flow is important for the rate of metabolism. Elimination half-life determines how long it takes to reach steady

state with the drug. As five half-lives are needed for steady state, it can be calculated that for morphine it will take from 10 to 20 hours to reach a steady state, whereas for methadone it may take between 20 and 650 hours.

Metabolism

Most opioids are metabolised in the liver by glucuronidation and/or demethylation (dealkylation) catalysed by CYP 450 isoenzymes, mainly 2D6 and 3A4. For at least morphine, hydromorphone and buprenorphine, glucuronidation is a major metabolic pathway. Human uridine disphosphate glucuronosyltransferases (e.g. UGT1A1 and UGT2B7) are polymorphic and inducible (e.g. by rifampicin and carbamazepine).

Box 20.4 Codeine: key pharmacokinetic facts

- Pro-drug – analgesic effect dependent on O-demethylation by CYP 2 D6 to **morphine**.
- CYP 2 D6 isoenzyme – polymorphic
- Ultrarapid metabolisers (*CYP2D6* gene duplication) – form higher amounts of morphine
  → **exaggerated opioid effect**
  May be life threatening even at doses of 75 mg especially if renal impairment
- Poor metabolisers (lack CYP2D6 activity) or CYP2D6 inhibition (e.g. paroxetine or quinidine) – poor analgesic effect despite high doses of codeine

---

Analgesia by codeine (Box 20.4) tramadol is reduced in poor metabolisers and if CYP2D6 is inhibited by, for example, paroxetine. Tramadol increases the availability of serotonin (and norepinephrine), whereas its main metabolite M1 (CYP2D6) is responsible for the opioid activity. The selective serotonin reuptake inhibitors (SSRIs), fluoxetine and paroxetine, are potent inhibitors of CYP2D6 and have a long half-life. The combination of either of these drugs with tramadol inhibits the metabolism of tramadol and increases its serotonergic activity, and potentially leads to serotonin syndrome (tremors, restlessness, fever and confusion). This interaction is also possible with other drugs that increase availability of serotonin, but the risk is smaller unless other drugs or pharmacogenetic factors cause an additional risk.

Table 20.2 Pharmacokinetic aspects of opioids.

Opioid	Terminal half-life (h)	Clearance (l/min)	Oral bio-availability (%)	Main metabolic pathway with	Active metabolites
Morphine	2–4	0.8–1.2	19–47	UGT1A1;2B7	M6G
Methadone	4–130	0.1–0.3	60–90	CYP 3A4/5;2D6;1A2;2B6;2C19	No
Fentanyl	4–8	0.7–1.5	<2/90 (TD)	CYP 3A4/5	No
Oxycodone	3.5 ± 0.8	0.4–1.1	40–130	CYP 3A4/5;2D6	Oxymorphone
Hydromorphone	2–4	0.4	35–80	UGT1A1;2B7	No
Codeine	3–4	0.6–0.9	60–90	CYP 2D6;3A4/5	Morphine
Tramadol	5–6	0.5–0.7	68–75	CYP 2D6;3A4/5	M1 (O-demethyltramadol)
Tapentadol	4.3 ± 0.8	1.5 ± 0.2	32	UGT1A6;UGT1A9;UGT2B7	No
Buprenorphine	20–25		(SL)	CYP3A4/5 & UGT1A1;2B7	

*SL = sublingual; TD = transdermal align="left"

CYP 3A4 is inducible. Induction of CYP 3A4/5 by rifampicin, carbamzepine or protease inhibitors (lopinavir/ritonavir) increases metabolism of methadone and thus reduces its efficacy. Higher doses of methadone are needed to maintain analgesia. On the other hand, inhibition of CYP 3A4/5 by drugs such as ciprofloxacin can lead to serious methadone toxicity. Similar interactions could be anticipated with buprenorphine, which is also a CYP 3A4/5 substrate.

Box 20.5 **Oxycodone: key pharmacokinetic facts**

- Main metabolite (90%) – N-demethylation by CYP 3A4 to noroxycodone (inactive)
- CYP3A4/5 inhibitors (e.g. itraconazole; grapefruit) increase the exposure to oxycodone
- Induction of CYP 3A4/5 (e.g. rifampicin) reduces efficacy
- 10% metabolism – O-demethylation by CYP 2D6 to oxymorphone (several times more potent)
- As very small amount of oxymorphone produced, blocking CYP2D6, unlikely to be clinically significant

---

Opioids undergo extensive hepatic biotransformation and their metabolites are excreted renally. If these metabolites are active (such as morphine-6-glucuronide), compromised renal function may lead to opioid toxicity (Box 20.6).

Box 20.6 **Opioids in renal failure**

In patients with significantly reduced renal function:

- lipophilic opioids that do not have active metabolites, such as buprenorphine, fentanyl and methadone, should be considered
- hydrophilic opioids like morphine and codeine that also have active metabolites should be avoided
- tramadol, hydromorphone and oxycodone can only be used with caution and close monitoring of the patients

---

Treatment of opioid-induced adverse effects

Acute administration of opioids can cause a wide range of adverse effects (Figure 20.4). Pain stimulates the respiratory centre whereas opioids depress it. Respiratory depression does not occur if titration of the opioid dose is successful against pain. Patients who have central sleep apnoea have increased sensitivity to opioid-induced respiratory depression. In the absence of pain, tolerance usually develops to opioid-induced respiratory depression. Respiratory depression, like all opioid-mediated effects, can be reversed with opioid-receptor antagonists like naloxone.

Nausea and vomiting are common opioid-induced adverse effects. Their mechanisms and treatment options are shown in Box 20.7.

Box 20.7 **Mechanisms and treatment of opioid-induced nausea and vomiting**

Nausea and vomiting are often the dose-limiting adverse effects of opioids. Opioids can cause emesis by direct stimulation of the chemoreceptor trigger zone (CTZ) or the vestibular apparatus, and through inhibition of gut motility. The CTZ is stimulated by opioid receptor activation. Butyrophenones such as haloperidol and droperidol act as antiemetics by blocking D_2 receptors. The vestibular apparatus is stimulated directly by opioids, and the sensory input to the vomiting centre occurs via the histamine H_1 and cholinergic ACh_m pathways. This explains why antihistamines and anticholinergic agents are effective against movement-induced nausea. Inhibition of gut motility causes emesis through serotonergic signalling to the vomiting centre. This can be blocked by $5HT_3$-receptor antagonists.

Opioids can also cause hallucinations and nightmares. Reducing the dose or changing the opioid can help. Butyrophenones can reduce this adverse effect.

Itching is usually an opioid receptor mediated effect that can be prevented with a small dose of an opioid antagonist. Morphine can also cause itching through histamine release. Sweating is a difficult-to-treat adverse effect of opioid therapy, particularly fentanyl.

Tolerance does not usually develop to constipation, which is a major problem, particularly in long-term opioid administration. As opioids cause constipation mainly through peripheral opioid receptors, constipation can be prevented by blocking peripheral opioid receptors in the gut. This can be achieved with an opioid antagonist that does not penetrate the blood–brain barrier (methylnaltrexone) or that is efficiently metabolised during first-pass metabolism

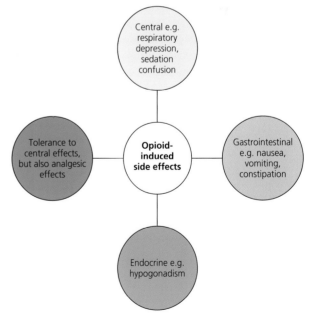

Figure 20.4 Opioid-induced adverse effects. Tolerance can develop to analgesia and all central adverse effects (but not to constipation, which is mainly a peripheral effect.

through liver (naloxone). These are expenses drugs and they should be used only if cheaper laxatives such as Na-picosulphate and lactulose are not effective enough.

Opioids have significant effects on the endocrine system. The effects are reversible after acute use but can persist and may cause serious symptoms if they are not diagnosed and treated in chronic opioid administration. Long-term opioid therapy can cause hypogonadism via central suppression of hypothalamic secretion of gonadotropin-releasing hormone, decreased pituitary luteinizing hormone, adrenal dehydroepiandrosterone and testosterone, decreased oestradiol and progesterone in women, and decreased testicular testosterone in men. Symptoms of opioid-induced hypogonadism include loss of libido, infertility, fatigue, depression, anxiety, loss of muscle strength and mass, osteoporosis, impotence and menstrual irregularities. Monitoring of hormone levels and hormone supplementation when indicated should be considered in chronic opioid therapy.

Conclusions

Good understanding of pain and pharmacology of opioids is necessary for the effective and safe use of opioids to manage chronic pain. Opioids are very effective analgesics but also have a number of significant adverse effects. There is limited evidence for their efficacy in long-term use and their benefit in individual patients should be reviewed regularly.

Further reading

Avouac, J, Gossec, L, Dougados, M (2007) Efficacy and safety of opioids for osteoarthritis: a meta-analysis of randomized controlled trials. *Osteo Arthritis and Cartilage*, **15**, 957–965.

British Pain Society with Royal College of Psychiatrists and Royal College of General Practitioners. http://britishpainsociety.org/pub professional.htm (accessed 12 December 2011).

Butler, SF, Budman, SH, Fernandez, KC, Houle, B, Benoit, C, Katz, N & Jamison, RN (2007) Development and validation of the Current Opioid Misuse Measure. *Pain*, **130**, 144–156.

Chou, R, Fanciullo, GJ, Fine, PG, Adler, JA, Ballantyne, JC, Davies, P, et al. (2009) Clinical guidelines for the use of chronic opioid therapy in chronic noncancer pain. *J Pain*, **10**, 113–130.

Dean, M (2004) Opioids in renal failure. *J Pain Symptom Manag*, **28**, 497–504.

Furlan, AD, Sandoval, JA, Mailis-Gagnon, A & Tunks, E (2006) Opioids for chronic noncancer pain: a meta-analysis of effectiveness and side effects. *Can Med Assoc J*, **174**, 1589–1594.

Jamison, RN, Ross, EL, Michna, E, Chen, LQ, Holcomb, C & Wasan, AD (2010) Substance misuse treatment for high-risk chronic pain patients on opioid therapy: a randomized study. *Pain*, **150**, 390–400.

Kalso, E, Allan, L, Dellemijn, PLI, Faura, CC, Ilias, WK, Jensen, TS, et al. (2003) Recommendations for using opioids in chronic non-cancer pain. *Eur J Pain*, **7**, 381–386.

Kalso, E, Edwards, J, Moore, RA & McQuay, HJ (2004) Opioids in chronic non-cancer pain. A systematic review. *Pain*, **112**, 372–380.

Kress, HG (2010) Tapentadol and its two mechanisms of action: is there a new pharmacological class of centrally-acting analgesics on the horizon? *Eur J Pain*, **14**, 781–783.

Martell, BA, O'Connor, PG, Kerns, RD, Becker, WC, Morales, KH, Kosten, TR & Flellin, DA (2007) Systematic review: Opioid treatment for chronic back pain: Prevalence, efficacy, and association with addiction. *Ann Intern Med*, **146**, 116–127.

McNicol, E, Boyce, DB, Schumann, R & Carr, D (2008) Efficacy and safety of mu-opioid antagonists in the treatment of opioid-induced bowel dysfunction: Systematic review and meta-analysis of randomized controlled trials. *Pain Medicine*, **9**, 634–659.

Niscola, P, Scaramucci, L, Vischini, G, Giovannini, M, Ferrannini, M, Massa, P, et al. (2010) The use of major analgesics in patients with renal dysfunction. *Curr Drug Targets*, **11**, 752–758.

Turk, DC, Swanson, KS & Gatchel, RJ (2008) Predicting opioid misuse by chronic pain patients: a systematic review and literature synthesis. *Clin J Pain*, **24**, 497–508.

Index

Numbers in *italics* refer to figures; numbers in **bold** refer to tables.

ALSO AVAILABLE

ABC of Adolescence
Russell Viner
2005 | 9780727915740 | 56 PAGES | £26.99/US$39.95/€34.90/AU$54.95

ABC of Allergies
Stephen R. Durham
1998 | 9780727912367 | 65 PAGES | £29.99/US$49.95/€38.90/AU$59.95

ABC of Antithrombotic Therapy
Gregory Y.H. Lip & Andrew D. Blann
2003 | 9780727917713 | 67 PAGES | £24.99/US$39.95/€32.90/AU$49.95

ABC of Arterial and Venous Disease, 2nd Edition
Richard Donnelly & Nick J.M. London
2009 | 9781405178891 | 120 PAGES | £29.99/US$52.95/€38.90/AU$59.95

ABC of Brain Stem Death, 2nd Edition
Christopher Pallis & D.H. Harley
1996 | 9780727902450 | 55 PAGES | £29.99/US$52.95/€38.90/AU$59.95

ABC of Breast Diseases, 3rd Edition
J. Michael Dixon
2005 | 9780727918284 | 120 PAGES | £32.99/US$56.95/€42.90/AU$67.95

ABC of Burns
Shehan Hettiaratchy, Remo Papini & Peter Dziewulski
2004 | 9780727917874 | 56 PAGES | £24.99/US$39.95/€32.90/AU$49.95

ABC of Child Protection, 4th Edition
Sir Roy Meadow, Jacqueline Mok & Donna Rosenberg
2007 | 9780727918178 | 120 PAGES | £32.99/US$56.95/€42.90/AU$67.95

ABC of Clinical Electrocardiography, 2nd Edition
Francis Morris, William Brady & John Camm
2008 | 9781405170642 | 112 PAGES | £32.99/US$54.95/€42.90/AU$67.95

ABC of Clinical Genetics, 3rd Edition
Helen M. Kingston
2002 | 9780727916273 | 120 PAGES | £29.99/US$54.95/€38.90/AU$59.95

ABC of Clinical Haematology, 3rd Edition
Drew Provan
2007 | 9781405153539 | 112 PAGES | £32.99/US$56.95/€42.90/AU$67.95

ABC of Colorectal Diseases, 2nd Edition
David Jones
1998 | 9780727911056 | 110 PAGES | £32.99/US$56.95/€42.90/AU$67.95

ABC of Complementary Medicine, 2nd Edition
Catherine Zollman, Andrew Vickers & Janet Richardson
2008 | 9781405136570 | 58 PAGES | £27.99/US$44.95/€35.90/AU$57.95

ABC of Conflict and Disaster
Anthony Redmond, Peter F. Mahoney, James Ryan, Cara Macnab & Lord David Owen
2005 | 9780727917263 | 80 PAGES | £24.99/US$39.95/€32.90/AU$49.95

ABC of Dermatology, 5th Edition
Paul K. Buxton & Rachael Morris-Jones
2009 | 9781405170659 | 224 PAGES | £32.99/US$55.95/€42.90/AU$67.95

ABC of Ear, Nose and Throat, 5th Edition
Harold S. Ludman & Patrick Bradley
2007 | 9781405136563 | 120 PAGES | £32.99/US$56.95/€42.90/AU$67.95

ABC of Eating Disorders
Jane Morris
2008 | 9780727918437 | 80 PAGES | £24.99/US$39.95/€32.90/AU$49.95

ABC of Emergency Differential Diagnosis
Francis Morris & Alan Fletcher
2009 | 9781405170635 | 96 PAGES | £29.99/US$52.95/€38.90/AU$59.95

ABC of Emergency Radiology, 2nd Edition
Otto Chan
2007 | 9780727915283 | 144 PAGES | £33.99/US$56.95/€43.90/AU$67.95

ABC of Eyes, 4th Edition
Peng T. Khaw, Peter Shah & Andrew R. Elkington
2004 | 9780727916594 | 104 PAGES | £30.99/US$52.95/€39.90/AU$62.95

ABC of the First Year, 6th Edition
Bernard Valman & Roslyn Thomas
2009 | 9781405180375 | 136 PAGES | £29.99/US$52.95/€38.90/AU$59.95

ABC of Geriatric Medicine
Nicola Cooper, Kirsty Forrest & Graham Mulley
2009 | 9781405169424 | 88 PAGES | £24.99/US$41.95/€32.90/AU$49.95

ABC of Headache
Anne MacGregor & Alison Frith
2008 | 9781405170666 | 88 PAGES | £22.99/US$39.95/€29.90/AU$47.95

ABC of Health Informatics
Frank Sullivan & Jeremy Wyatt
2006 | 9780727918505 | 56 PAGES | £24.99/US$39.95/€32.90/AU$49.95

ABC of Heart Failure, 2nd Edition
Russell C. Davis, Michael K. Davies & Gregory Y.H. Lip
2006 | 9780727916440 | 72 PAGES | £24.99/US$39.95/€32.90/AU$49.95

ABC of Hypertension, 5th Edition
Gareth Beevers, Gregory Y.H. Lip & Eoin O'Brien
2007 | 9781405130615 | 88 PAGES | £29.99/US$49.95/€38.90/AU$59.95

ABC of Kidney Disease
David Goldsmith, Satish Jayawardene & Penny Ackland
2007 | 9781405136754 | 96 PAGES | £32.99/US$54.95/€42.90/AU$67.95

ABC of Labour Care
Geoffrey Chamberlain, Philip Steer & Luke Zander
1999 | 9780727914156 | 60 PAGES | £23.99/US$37.95/€30.90/AU$47.95

ABC of Liver, Pancreas and Gall Bladder
Ian Beckingham
2001 | 9780727915313 | 64 PAGES | £23.99/US$37.95/€30.90/AU$47.95

ABC of Lung Cancer
Ian Hunt, Martin M. Muers & Tom Treasure
2009 | 9781405146524 | 64 PAGES | £24.99/US$39.95/€32.90/AU$49.95

ABC of Major Trauma, 3rd Edition
Peter Driscoll, David Skinner & Richard Earlam
1999 | 9780727913784 | 192 PAGES | £29.99/US$52.95/€38.90/AU$59.95

ABC of Medical Law
Lorraine Corfield, Ingrid Granne & William Latimer-Sayer
2009 | 9781405176286 | 64 PAGES | £23.99/US$37.95/€30.90/AU$47.95

ABC of Mental Health, 2nd Edition
Teifion Davies & Tom Craig
2009 | 9780727916396 | 128 PAGES | £30.99/US$49.95/€39.90/AU$62.95

ABC of Monitoring Drug Therapy
Jeffrey Aronson, M. Hardman & D.J.M. Reynolds
1993 | 9780727907912 | 46 PAGES | £24.99/US$39.95/€32.90/AU$49.95

ABC of Nutrition, 4th Edition
A. Stewart Truswell
2003 | 9780727916648 | 152 PAGES | £29.99/US$52.95/€38.90/AU$59.95

ABC of Obesity
Naveed Sattar & Mike Lean
2007 | 9781405136747 | 64 PAGES | £24.99/US$37.94/€32.90/AU$49.95

ABC of One to Seven, 5th Edition
Bernard Valman
2009 | 9781405181051 | 168 PAGES | £30.99/US$49.95/€39.90/AU$62.95

ABC of Oral Health
Crispian Scully
2000 | 9780727915511 | 41 PAGES | £23.99/US$37.95/€30.90/AU$47.95

ABC of Palliative Care, 2nd Edition
Marie Fallon & Geoffrey Hanks
2006 | 9781405130790 | 96 PAGES | £28.99/US$49.95/€37.90/AU$57.95

ABC of Patient Safety
John Sandars & Gary Cook
2007 | 9781405156929 | 64 PAGES | £26.99/US$44.95/€34.90/AU$54.95

ABC of Practical Procedures
Tim Nutbeam & Ron Daniels
2009 | 9781405185950 | 144 PAGES | £29.99/US$47.95/€38.90/AU$59.95

ABC of Preterm Birth
William McGuire & Peter Fowlie
2005 | 9780727917638 | 56 PAGES | £24.99/US$39.95/€32.90/AU$49.95

ABC of Psychological Medicine
Richard Mayou, Michael Sharpe & Alan Carson
2003 | 9780727915566 | 72 PAGES | £26.99/US$39.95/€34.90/AU$54.95

ABC of Resuscitation, 5th Edition
Michael Colquhoun, Anthony Handley & T.R. Evans
2003 | 9780727916693 | 111 PAGES | £32.99/US$56.95/€42.90/AU$67.95

ABC of Rheumatology, 4th Edition
Ade Adebajo
2009 | 9781405170680 | 192 PAGES | £30.99/US$47.95/€39.90/AU$62.95

ABC of Sepsis
Ron Daniels & Tim Nutbeam
2009 | 9781405181945 | 104 PAGES | £29.99/US$49.95/€38.90/AU$59.95

ABC of Sexual Health, 2nd Edition
John Tomlinson
2004 | 9780727917591 | 96 PAGES | £29.99/US$49.95/€38.90/AU$59.95

ABC of Skin Cancer
Sajjad Rajpar & Jerry Marsden
2008 | 9781405162197 | 80 PAGES | £24.99/US$44.95/€32.90/AU$49.95

ABC of Smoking Cessation
John Britton
2004 | 9780727918185 | 56 PAGES | £22.99/US$37.95/€29.90/AU$47.95

ABC of Spinal Disorders
Andrew Clarke, Alwyn Jones, Michael O'Malley & Robert McLaren
2009 | 9781405170697 | 72 PAGES | £23.99/US$37.95/€30.90/AU$47.95

ABC of Sports and Exercise Medicine, 3rd Edition
Gregory Whyte, Mark Harries & Clyde Williams
2005 | 9780727918130 | 136 PAGES | £32.99/US$59.95/€42.90/AU$67.95

ABC of Subfertility
Peter Braude & Alison Taylor
2004 | 9780727915344 | 64 PAGES | £23.99/US$37.95/€30.90/AU$47.95

ABC of Transfusion, 4th Edition
Marcela Contreras
2009 | 9781405156462 | 128 PAGES | £29.99/US$52.95/€38.90/AU$59.95

ABC of Tubes, Drains, Lines and Frames
Adam Brooks, Peter F. Mahoney & Brian Rowlands
2008 | 9781405160148 | 88 PAGES | £24.99/US$39.95/€32.90/AU$49.95

ABC of the Upper Gastrointestinal Tract
Robert Logan, Adam Harris, J.J. Misiewicz & J.H. Baron
2002 | 9780727912664 | 54 PAGES | £24.99/US$39.95/€32.90/AU$49.95

ABC of Wound Healing
Joseph E. Grey & Keith G. Harding
2006 | 9780727916952 | 56 PAGES | £24.99/US$39.95/€32.90/AU$49.95

For more information on any of our medical books, please visit **www.wiley.com/go/medicine**